Applied Immunological Concepts

Contents

Preface

Rapid and significant developments occurring in recent years have modified and enlarged the scope of the science of immunology. Nursing practitioners and students frequently voice concern regarding their lack of comprehension of these developments. Immunology is an area of complex theory and speculation; almost daily we are presented with new developments. The research and resulting literature appear somewhat awesome to the individual who has not been regularly immersed in the study of immunology. A structure of essential concepts is necessary if one expects to assimilate and utilize various theoretical frameworks and comprehend relevant data.

The purpose of this book is to describe current concepts of immunological science. The application of immunology in health promotion and health maintenance as well as related nursing interventions will be discussed. Immunological terminology, although descriptive and valuable, can provide the nonimmunologist with a basis for confusion and frustration. To understand the concepts a new vocabulary must be developed. Thus, terminology is defined as it is introduced to facilitate an understanding by the reader.

Nursing is a health-oriented profession with its emphasis on providing for the achievement of one's maximum developmental potential. Immunological competence is learned throughout life.

It is in itself a developmental process. At birth the human organism has a genetically determined self, which is further refined by
the individual's contact with antigens (immunological stressors)
in the environment. The inability to develop immunological competence can alter man's developmental process, as well as his
potential for existence itself.

It therefore seems fitting that a presentation of immunological
concepts for nurses be done with a developmental framework. We
will attempt a discussion of the gross and microscopic anatomy
and physiology of the system, considering genetic determination
and development of the response, with emphasis on changes as
they relate to both physiological and environmental stimulation.

Introduction

The purpose of describing the gross and microscopic anatomy of the immunological system is to illustrate the relationship of structure to function, both normal and dysfunctional. Unlike the format of textbooks of anatomy and physiology, which should be consulted for finer details, this book only discusses the gross and microscopic components with clinical implications. This should provide a comprehensive understanding of both the form and function of the immunological system and a normal base from which variations can be interpreted.

At this point in time a nursing practice model for immunological concepts appears only as a glimmer visible through the application of the nursing process to the multiple specialty areas. The nature of practice is not limited to a single area of specialization. It is our belief that one day immunological principles will influence all levels of nursing practice.

The major purpose of this book is to assist the nurse working with a patient whose condition imposes immunological implications to implement effective, efficient, and coordinated programs of diagnostics, therapeutics, and patient education. The components of the nursing process—assessment, diagnosis, and planning— are all basic to activating this conceptual base. The future holds the practice components of implementation and evaluation.

We have taken what is known in the field of immunology relevant to nursing practice and woven these concepts into a general functional nursing model. The establishment of a specific practice model requires extensive efforts on the part of nursing practitioners. The skills of prediction and prevention are close at hand given the right amount of effort and priority setting by all those concerned with this field.

The number of references used to prepare the text was exhaustive, to say the least. In the initial draft, all references were noted in the body of the text; however, this made the reading of an already complicated text almost an unpleasant task. Therefore, all references are listed at the conclusion of subject matter components; no footnotes appear in the text. Some reference lists were appropriately placed at the conclusion of chapters; others follow individual sections of chapters. The rationale used to determine placement consisted of localization of resources proximal to the concept considered, enabling the reader to identify authors who have commented further on areas of the text which have stimulated their desire to investigate these subjects in greater depth. You may also note that the number of references from nursing literature is almost negligible. This is not an omission, but a reflection of reality at this point in time.

The comments of the reader related to this format and consideration of the subject are welcomed by the authors.

Applied Immunological Concepts

CHAPTER ONE

A Conceptual
Model-Related Theory

A model can be defined as a relatively simple depiction in symbolic terms of the structure of a system. The model is composed of concepts that usually give reference to the structures and processes of a system. The model does not reflect the total reality; rather, it explains reality in an abstract, comprehensible manner.

Today, conceptual models are being used in practice and in education not only to direct function, but to identify critical content essential to the understanding of various subjects. The model we have constructed for the immunological system identifies the structural components of the system, the processes that the system carries out, and its functional capacities.

Although the model is presented initially, its usefulness is not complete until one understands the content related to each concept. One must start with the most basic concepts and move to the abstract. The model provides a structure to view relationships, sources of stress, and areas for further investigation. Results of further research can be incorporated within the concepts to which they apply and model alterations developed accordingly; thus a flexible foundation for the growth of knowledge is provided.

The model also allows one to note the place where stressors can occur. The realization that stressors affect all segments above their point of impact permits identification of variables and areas where

1

needs may arise, thus indicating points of intervention. When combined within a practice framework, the model assures a scientific, rational, organized approach to nursing diagnosis of health problems associated with the immunological system.

THE MODEL

In man, a competent immunological system evolves from appropriate interactions between cell populations. Conceptually, the interactions result in an effective physiological defense mechanism. Thus, the model itself is an interactional defense system. The system is illustrated in Figure 1. Immunological stresses in the environment are *recognized* as they penetrate the boundaries of the human system; the human system *responds* with three levels of defense.

The defense mechanism consists of local barriers, the inflamma-

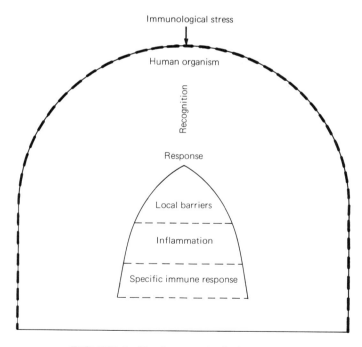

FIGURE 1 The immunological system.

tion process, and the specific immune response. One or all of these levels of action can be initiated following the recognition phase. Immunological stress is antigenic in nature and is stress perceived by the human organism as nonself or foreign to human system. The human organism has the innate capability to recognize cell populations and protein substances which compose the body systems. When cell populations and protein substances not components of the original system are introduced, they are recognized as nonself and a defense initiated.

The defense has both gross and microscopic components at both the recognition and response level. These components are activated by immunological stress, and the resulting defense is related to the integrity of these structures as well as the innate and acquired sensitivities of the system.

DEVELOPMENT OF THE CELL POPULATIONS

During embryological development the fertilized ovum, a unicellular organism, has the potential to differentiate and develop multiple types of cell populations. This potential includes the ability to develop cell populations that perform the specific functions of the immunological system. Figure 2 depicts the development of the cell populations of the immunological system as well as the regulators of this developmental process.

Stem cells from the differentiating fertilized ovum have the

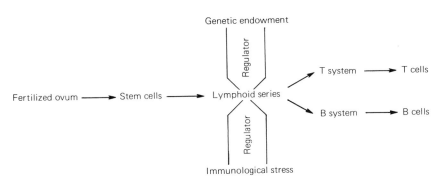

FIGURE 2 Cell population development.

potential to develop the cells of the lymphoid series. The lymphoid series can further differentiate into the T cell and B cell components of the immunological system. This differentiation is regulated by genetic endowment and later exposure to immunological stress. The resulting cell populations have the capacity to recognize and react to immunological stress. They act to either initiate or support other populations of cells in response to immunological stress.

Immunological stress is therefore an internal or external threat to the ecology of the human system. Most immunological stressors are called antigens and are substances capable of initiating an immunological response. Keep in mind that immunological stressors are perceived by the human system as nonself and that this perception is related to the integrity of the total system as well as its innate and acquired sensitivities.

IMMUNOLOGICAL STRESS

There are a broad host of microorganisms in man, many of which exhibit a symbiotic or close association with him. Some, known as the normal flora, are beneficial. Each microorganism has the capacity to invade the host, to resist phagocytosis, and to secrete toxins. The environment and man's genetic structure, as well as multiple insect vectors, may act as immunological stressors on a complex delicately balanced relationship (Fig. 3). A competitive

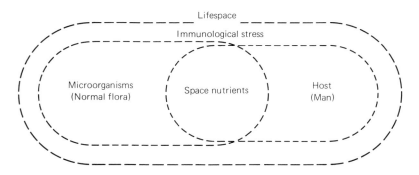

FIGURE 3 Host-microorganism ecological system.

relationship for space and nutrients exists between man and his natural flora of microorganisms. Man, the host, provides barriers against stressors, such as the skin, mucous membranes, and conjunctiva. However, contamination can occur directly through inhalation, ingestion, and via venereal routes. Indirect contamination may result from contact with inanimate objects. Malnutrition can result in changes in barrier integrity, production of body fluids, and enzyme antagonists. Phagocytic function and antibody formation itself may be altered, resulting in altered intestinal flora. Reduction of oxygen availability due to inadequate blood supply decreases reduction potentials of human tissues. This anaerobic environment will promote increased growth of organisms in wounds in which growth of anaerobic organisms normally would be controlled by local mechanisms.

Recognition: Genetic Endowment

It appears that the ability to develop cell populations with specific susceptibility to respond to antigenic stimulation is genetically determined. This determination is an energetically explored area of immunobiology. A complete understanding of the most basic mechanism controlling the ability to distinguish self from nonself has the potential to control immunological activity. Since this is the most basic determinant to immunological activity, it is basic to the recognition arm of the immunological system. Any stress to the genetic determinants will most certainly effect all levels of system function.

The stem cells are the cells of the primitive blood islands and the yolk sac of the embryo. They differentiate into the cells of the lymphatic and hematopoietic systems. The fetal liver is the source of the stem cell in fetal life, and the bone marrow is responsible for the production of stem cells throughout life. As mentioned in the previous paragraph the stem cell receives a code for differentiation from the genes; in addition it is responsive to the environment.

The cell populations are derived from either the cellular or humoral arms of the immunological system. The cellular arm is composed of T cells which provide cellular immunity. The humoral arm is composed of plasma cells (B cells) which secrete immuno-

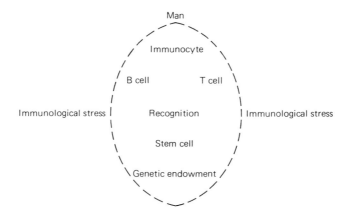

FIGURE 4   Immune response resulting from immunological stress.

globulins providing specific antibodies. These cells cooperate in the formation of the final effector of the specific immune response—the immunocyte.

The term *immunocyte* is used to describe the cell that initiates the sequence of events following exposure to immunological stress (an antigen to which the organism is susceptible). The specific immune response resulting from recognition of immunological stress is depicted in Figure 4.

Response

There are basically three levels of a defense response: local barriers, inflammation, and the specific immune response. Local barriers, such as skin, conjunctiva, and mucous membrane provide both mechanical and chemical defenses. The inflammatory response culminates in phagocytosis. The inflammatory process begins after invader organisms pass the local barrier defense level. It is characterized by blood vessel dilitation and increased vascular permeability. This results in additional plasma containing leukocytes and erythrocytes entering into the extracellular space. The granulocytic polymorphoneutrophils (PMNS), pass between endothelial cells of blood capillaries into the site of injury. These are the earliest phagocytic cells. The monocytic phase follows. Plasma containing serum, immunoglobulins, complement, and fibrinogen enter the injury site. If antibody activity for invader organisms is present, the antibody coats the antigenic invader and facilitates engulfment of the organism by phagocytosis. Fibrin is deposited close to the injury site.

If the inflammatory response is inadequate to contain the invading organism, the organism is transported to the lymph nodes where it is again processed in a similar manner, and the specific immune response is initiated. The reticuloendothelial macrophages phagocytize bacteria that have been washed from afferent lymphatics. This stimulates inflammation of the lymphatics. Filtration capability is therefore increased. Sinus channels in lymph nodes become filled with polymorphoneutrophils and monocytes. Eventually the regional node is penetrated. If its filtration capabilities are inadequate, invading organisms enter the thoracic duct and the bloodstream. It is via this route that organisms can invade any part of the body and a specific immune response is initiated.

The specific immune response results in disintegration of intact microorganisms or their toxic by-products by host cells. This response may be humoral (antibody mediated) or cell mediated. The humoral and/or cell mediated response potentiates the effectiveness of the phagocytic cells.

IMMUNITY OR IMMUNOLOGICAL RESPONSE

Immunity is an ability of the human system to deal effectively with immunological stress. Immunity has been classified as innate (genetic endowment), acquired (which is either natural or artificial), and adoptive. Since innate immunity is genetically endowed, it is a constant for a specific species and cannot be transferred to other species.

Acquired natural immunity can evolve actively through contracting a disease and recovering, or passively from one's mother via an intrauterine route prior to birth or from IgG present in colostrum and breast milk. Acquired artificial immunity is developed actively after vaccination or immunization, or passively when one receives serum from an immune individual.

Adoptive immunity results from the transfer of factors from lymphoid cells of immune humans to recipients. It is an experimental procedure but appears to be a means by which immunity can be provided. The concept of adoptive immunity promises to be of great interest and importance in the future.

Functional Capacity of the Response

During the immune response an immunological stressor (antigen) interacts with a cell by means of an attraction between a surface receptor on the cell which is attracted to the specific antigenic group. The two cells interact once and produce a proliferation of cells that can act with similar specificity or function in the future to recognize similar antigens (memory cells).

Amplification

It is possible for the immunological response to be amplified. Amplification in these situations is the sum of responses initiated by a specific immune response that results in an additional inflammatory response.

Tolerance

There are times when the immunological system is unable to respond to antigenic immunological stress. The inability to respond to antigenic material in an otherwise immunologically intact individual is termed immunological tolerance.

SUMMARY

The immunological system of man is conceptually a defense mechanism, acting through the genetic and environmentally controlled development of specific cell populations. The basic interactional units are a recognition and response phase that can be amplified by the stimulation of associated support systems.

The human organism acts as a host microorganism ecological

system utilizing the immunological system to defend against immunological stress. The defense itself has three distinct, although interactive levels: local barriers, the inflammation process, and the specific immune response. If an organism with an otherwise intact immunological system is unable to mount a defense, it is said to exhibit immunological tolerance.

Hopefully, this broad conceptual approach to a complicated system will assist the reader in integrating the later concepts in this volume. The reader should refer to the original model and reflect on the specifics contained in later chapters.

SUGGESTED READINGS

Braun W: Bacterial Genetics, 2nd ed. Philadelphia, Saunders, 1965

Davis BQ et al.: Microbiology, 2nd ed. Hagerstown, Md, Harper & Row, 1973

Hozzard ME, Kergin DJ: An overview of system theory. Nurs Clin North Am 6:3, September 1971

Gottlieb AA, Waldman SR: The multiple function of macrophages in immunity. CRC Crit Rev Microbiol 2:321, 1972

Katz DH, Benacerrof B: The regulatory influence of activated cells on B cell responses to antigen. Adv Immunol 15:1, 1972

McDevitt HO, Benacerraf B: Genetic control of specific immune responses. Adv Immunol 11:31, 1969

Nossal CTV, Ada CL: Antigens, Lymphoid Cells and the Immune Response. New York, Academic, 1971

Playpair JHL: Cell cooperation in the immune response. Clin Exp Immun 8:839–856, 1971

Riehl JR, Roy Sr. C: Conceptual Models for Nursing Practice. New York, Appleton, 1974

Sela M: Antigenicity: some molecular aspects. Science 166:1365, 1969

Silverstein AM, Prendergast RA: Lymphogenesis, immunogenesis, and the generation of immunological diversity. In Sterzl J, Riha I (eds): Developmental Aspects of Antibody Formation and Structure. New York, Academic, 1971

Sterzl J et al.: Developmental Aspects of Immunity. Immun 61:337–459, 1967

Unanoe ER, Ceroltini JC: The function of macrophages in the immune response. Seminars Hemat 7:225–248, 1970

CHAPTER TWO

The Structures
and Functions of
the Immunological System

Two systems of immunity are responsible for protecting the body against the hazards of foreign antigens, infection, or even cancer. One is the cell-mediated immune response (T system), which is composed of a large number of cells (10^{12}) known as T lymphocytes. It combats fungi and most viruses, and it initiates the process by which organ transplants and tumors are rejected. The other system is the humoral system (B system). It is composed of even a larger number (10^{20}) of protein molecules called antibodies which are secreted by specialized plasma lymphocytes (B cells). The humoral system is effective against bacteria and some viruses. The two mechanisms are distinct but not entirely independent.

Both components are composed of highly diversified cells derived from a single precursor, the stem cell. During embryogenesis the stem cells are found in the yolk sac of the fertilized ovum. The stem cells migrate to other recognized sites of hematopoietic development: the liver, spleen, and finally the bone marrow. The bone marrow is the major reservoir of stem cells in adult life. The stem cell under proper differentiation by its environment has the multipotential of developing into the granulocytes, the erythrocytes, the megakaryocytes, and the lymphocytes (Fig. 5). The lymphocyte provides the cellular basis for immunity. The lymphoid cells may differentiate into the thymic dependent lympho-

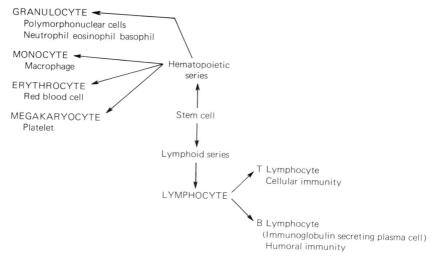

FIGURE 5 Multipotential development of the stem cell.

cyte (T cell) or the bone-marrow-dependent lymphocyte (plasma B cell) which secretes immunoglobulin (antibodies).

It is possible to differentiate the T and B cells on a morphological basis. The T cell has a flat, fairly smooth surface and the B cells have numerous projections on their surface. Research has developed a variety of ways to tag small lymphocytes in order to differentiate the two populations. It is well recognized that the primitive precursor for both populations is the stem cell (Fig. 5). Although distinct characteristics make it possible to identify the two systems as separate entities, it is also known that each cooperates with the other in the final process of defense against foreign invasion.

For the sake of clarity each system will be discussed separately, but the reader should always be mindful of the complexity of the defense process and its cooperative interactions. The presence of immunological stressors, i.e., antigens in the environment, and their recognition as foreign or nonself is responsible for the initiation of the immunological response of each system. Recall that an antigen is any substance that can stimulate the immune system. Natural antigens, largely made up of proteins and polysaccharides, have multiple surface reaction sites or antigen determinant sites, which are the points of interaction for the T and B system.

CELL-MEDIATED IMMUNOLOGICAL SYSTEM (CMI): T SYSTEM

Development of the T Cell Population

The cellular precursors of the lymphoid series undergo a very specific differentiation process. Early in development embryonic structures called the pharyngeal pouches migrate into the chest to form the thymus. Beginning about the eighth week of gestation in human life the blood-borne bone marrow stem cells enter the thymus. The immunological system is initially incapable of differentiating between self and nonself. It appears that the thymus and its humoral substances, e.g., thymosin play a relevant role in the development of "learning self." During the fetal period the differentiated T cell passes through the thymus where certain T cells are either paralyzed or eliminated. This developmental process results in the destruction of T cells that without thymic influence would have perceived components of the human organism as foreign. Thus self and nonself are recognized. This process also establishes the basis for life-long differentiation between self and nonself.

While the stem cells are residing in the thymus, they are converted into immunocompetent T cells. Hormones from the thymus promote maturation. After the lymphocyte leaves the thymus, the thymic hormones continue to exert thymic influence and maximize the potential of T cell function. Mature T cells emerge from the thymic medulla via the circulation; however, they are not restricted to the bloodstream and when not circulating reside in the lymphoid tissues. T cells are the major type of cell found in the lymph nodes, spleen, Peyer's patches, bone marrow, and intestinal mucosa. They are localized in specific thymic dependent areas such as the paracortex of the lymph nodes and the white pulp of the spleen.* After a short period of residency in lymphatic tissue areas, some of the cells enter the lymphatics and are returned to the circulation by way of the thoracic duct. These are called circulating T cells.

Noncirculating populations of T cells are subpopulations that

---

*There are three populations of T cells: circulating, noncirculating, and memory cells.

produce mediators or lymphokines and selectively migrate to inflammatory sites. The memory cells are another subpopulation of T cells and provide the ability for the T system to recognize antigens long after the initial exposure. These memory cells are radioresistant and can survive even after exposure to large doses of radiation therapy. The T lymphocytes are among the most rapidly proliferating cells in the body and have been identified with life spans up to 10 years.

Functional Specificity

Each cell has the capacity to recognize its particular antigenic determinant. Millions of antigenic determinants exist, and it seems that there are immunologically competent cells capable of recognizing each determinant. The nature of the antigen receptor on the T cell is not clearly understood, and speculation still surrounds many of the molecular events which take place.

T cells do not secrete antibodies but engage in combat as a T cell. They are capable of attack, inhibition, ingestion, destruction, or in some manner inactivate the offending antigen until the macrophages arrive.

Facilitating the Function of the CMI

LYMPHOKINES

To appreciate the functions of CMI one needs to look at the phenomena of lymphokines. In the presence of antigen the T lymphocyte is capable of inducing the production of lymphokines. Lymphokines are mediator substances that facilitate the immune response and bring about the destruction of the antigen. Identified lymphokines include chemotactic factor (CF), migratory inhibition factor (MIF), macrophage activation factor (MAF), blastogenic factor (BF), transfer factor (TF), lymphotoxin, and interferon.

Lymphokines are produced following a "killer" T cell-antigen interaction. Once the interaction has occurred, lymphokine

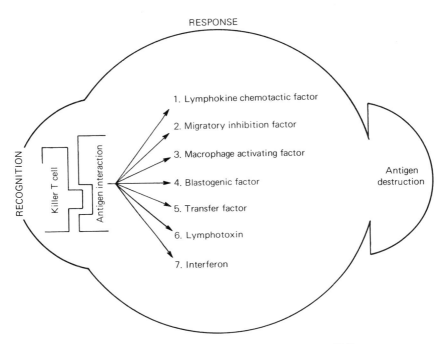

FIGURE 6 Facilitating the function of the CMI.

chemotactic factor is put into action. It is chemotactic (chemically attracted) for macrophages, eosinophils, and neutrophils. Chemotactic factor is largely responsible for promoting the migration of macrophages and sensitized T cells to the site of the antigen. The previously sensitized lymphocyte releases migratory inhibition factor (MIF), which prevents any further migration by the macrophage and thereby holds it at the site of the antigen. At the same time transfer factor begins its work of converting non-sensitized T cells to sensitized T cells, while blastogenic factor initiates cell growth (mitosis) of the sensitized T cell population. Macrophage activating factor (MAF) is activated and transforms local macrophages into intense phagocytes. Lymphotoxin assists the sensitized T cell in the direct destruction of the antigen by its ability to change the morphology and motility of the antigen resulting in rupture of the cell membrane. This process is depicted in Figure 6.

FUNCTIONS OF CELL-MEDIATED IMMUNITY

Defense

The CMI functions to defend the human organism against invasion by infectious agents, in the autoimmune response, in delayed hypersensitivity reactions, in transplant rejections, graft versus host reactions and surveillance against cancer. Each of the functions will be briefly discussed in this section and elaborated on in later chapters.

INFECTIOUS AGENTS

No general rule can be applied about the defense the CMI provides against infectious agents. Historically and experientially, CMI is known to play a major role in the defense against tuberculosis, measles, varicella, vaccinia, and *Candida*.

Individuals with defective CMI manifest an unusual susceptibility primarily to fungus and most viruses. Well-meaning immunization can lead to fatal infectious episodes for these individuals because they are unable to defend themselves against the stress of the infectious agent.

AUTOIMMUNE RESPONSE

Autoimmune disease occurs when the human organism perceives components of itself as antigenic or nonself and proceeds to destroy these components as if they were foreign substances. Both the T and B system are implicated. The point to be made is that the reactions result in harm to the individual rather than protection.

DELAYED HYPERSENSITIVITY REACTION

The classic example of delayed hypersensitivity is the skin reaction following intradermal innoculation or cutaneous exposure to the purified protein derivative (PPD) antigens. A peak reaction occurs between 48 and 72 hours. The major cellular component in the CMI reaction is the macrophage. Lymphokines are responsible for their presence. Generally speaking, cell-mediated hypersensitivities are not life threatening.

TRANSPLANT REJECTION (HOST VERSUS GRAFT)

The CMI plays a major role in organ transplant rejection. Observations have led to the conclusion that the transfer of sensitized cells that are antigenic to the human organism (e.g., animal sera) result in graft rejection.

GRAFT VERSUS HOST REACTIONS

If the CMI in the host is incompetent, a reverse of the host versus graft reaction can occur and is called a graft versus host reaction. In it the host is attacked. In this reaction the immunoincompetent host becomes the graft in response to the immunocompetent lymphocytes in the grafted tissue. These reactions are severe and often result in death.

SURVEILLANCE AGAINST CANCER

There is strong evidence that the T cell functions as the major cell component in the immune system's surveillance against cancer. It continually watches and destroys detected tumor cells. If surveillance fails, cancer results.

HUMORAL-MEDIATED IMMUNOLOGICAL SYSTEM (HMI): B SYSTEM

Up to this point we have considered only the role of the T system in providing a defense against immunological stress. The B system is composed of plasma cells that secrete antibodies. The substances also have a significant role in providing a defense against immunological stress. The plasma cell population secretes about 2000 identical protein antibody molecules per second. Each of the innumerable protein molecules is made up of peptide chains that form linear strings of a few hundred amino acids. Each antibody molecule is composed of two pairs of polypeptide chains which may be heavy or light chains depending on their length and molecular weight. Collectively they are called immunoglobulins. Parts of the immunoglobulin chains unfold and expose small patches or clefts (epitomes) on their surface, making them highly specific. Thus, the sequence of amino acids determines the class of immunoglobulin and, therefore, its biological role, whereas the arrangement of the clefts determines its specificity.

Patterns of Response

The immunoglobulins are the mediators of B system humoral-mediated immunity. They are present in the blood, exocrine secretions, and tissues. All immunoglobulins are serum proteins, but not all serum proteins are immunoglobulins.

Much of what is known about the B cell is based on an understanding of its products, the immunoglobulins. It appears that the B cell begins its development as a stem cell derived originally from the bone marrow and influenced in some way by the lymphoid tissue lining of the intestinal tract. In an attempt to bridge this gap of knowledge regarding the exact derivation and developmental progression of the B cell, most immunologists have subscribed to theoretical models. One such model is that of clonal selection. This model is divided into two stages: clonal development and clonal proliferation.

Stage I, clonal development, involves the conversion of stem cells into antigen-reactive B cells. This process consists of the genetic events that result in the synthesis of immunoglobulins. Immunoglobulin is then located on the cell membrane where its function is antigen recognition. A pair of genes determines the specificity of the B cell or the class of immunoglobulin it will produce. The B cell develops clones, i.e., a population of cells derived by asexual division from a single cell. The end result is the production of a clone of B cells genetically programmed to synthesize antibodies of a single immunoglobulin class with a single specificity.

Stage II, clonal proliferation, begins when Stage I cells with specific surface receptors enter the circulation. The order of entry of cells of the hypothetical clone occurs in an orderly sequence. When the new B cell first comes into contact with antigen, it is stimulated to proliferate and form memory cells or to differentiate into more antibody-producing plasma cells.

There are various mechanisms through which the humoral immune response is modulated. They consist of cooperative interactions with T cells and macrophages, feedback inhibition by circulating antibodies, and possibly many others. These mechanisms are believed to be operative during the stage of clonal proliferation.

Antibody production following exposure to an antigen can be evaluated by measuring the amount of antibody produced. On initial exposure the first immunoglobulin to respond is IgM. This response occurs in a time span of approximately six days. Around 10 to 14 days later IgG can also be detected. This initial response is considered a primary response. If a second exposure to the same antigen occurs at some later date, a minimal IgM response results, but much higher levels of IgG are seen. This is considered a secondary response (anamnestic response or memory phenomena). It results because some B cells remained which were already programmed to produce IgG in response to specific antigenic stimulation.

Antibodies produced during a secondary response are of a higher binding capacity (affinity) than those in the primary response. These cells bear surface receptors that are very precisely matched to the antigenic groupings on the antigen and are able to bind more firmly than cells with low-affinity antibodies. Moreover, exposure to small amounts of antigen stimulates high-affinity antibodies, and a large amount of antigen is needed to stimulate low-affinity antibodies. Immunoglobulins with high-affinity antibody will bind available antigen when low-affinity antigen is present, thus leaving the low-affinity antibody unbound. This is the proposed rationale behind the desensitization process. It is hypothesized that IgG, which is a high-affinity antibody, is bound to available antigen, leaving low-affinity IgE unbound and blocking the initiation of an allergic reaction, which is IgE mediated. This is also thought to be the effect of Rho-GAM in the Rh sensitive mother.

Immunoglobulins

To date, five classes of immunoglobulins in humans have been identified: IgG, IgM, IgA, IgD, and IgE. As previously stated the immunoglobulins are made of both heavy and light amino acid polypeptide chains. Physical and biological characteristics of the five major classes in man are summarized in Table 1. These characteristics provide the basis for identification of specific immunoglobulins, normal serum levels, and the expected rate of synthesis in the adult.

Characteristics of Immunoglobulins

IgG

IgG is the second immunoglobulin to respond to challenge by an antigen. It is probably the major immunoglobulin to respond in a secondary response. The half-life of IgG is about 25 days, the longest half-life of any plasma protein. IgG has four known subclasses: IgG_1, IgG_2, IgG_3, and IgG_4. It is the only immunoglobulin that has the ability to cross the placenta and therefore, it provides a major line of the defense against infection for the first few weeks of an infant's life. IgG levels appear to be enhanced in breast-fed infants, probably due to the presence of IgG in colostrum and breast milk. IgG diffuses readily into extravascular body spaces and bears the major burden of neutralizing bacterial toxins. It also has the ability to bind to microorganisms, enhancing the process of phagocytosis. IgG antibodies can also coat target cells, which prepares the cell for killing.

There is a regulatory mechanism that controls the synthesis of IgG. This mechanism is a response to feedback regarding existing levels of circulating IgG and is also responsive to stimulation by antigen.

IgM

IgM is the first antibody produced in response to primary antigenic stimulation. IgM antibodies are extremely efficient as agglutinating and cytolytic agents and found primarily (75 percent) in the intravascular circulation. IgM possesses opsonin and complement-fixing properties, accounting for its aggulutinating and cytolytic functions.

IgA

IgA occurs both in the circulation and body secretions. Secretory IgA is similar to circulating IgA, but it is accompanied by a trans-

TABLE 1 Physical and Biological Characteristics of the Five Major Classes of Immunoglobulin.

	IgG	IgA	IgM	IgD	IgE
Normal/serum (mg/100 ml)	800–1,680	140–420	50–190	0.3–40	0.0001–0.0007
Mean–adult	1,200	300	150	3	0.03
Percent of total	70–80	13–16	5–10	1.0	0.002
Valance for binding	2	2	5–10	?	2
Molecular weight	150,000	180–500,000	900,000	180,000	200,000
Synthesis rate	25 mg/kg/day		7 mg/kg/day		

port piece. IgA appears selectively in seromucous secretions such as tears, saliva, nasal secretions, sweat, colostrum, and secretions of the lung and gastrointestinal tract. It defends exposed body surfaces against the invasion of microorganisms. IgA is synthesized locally in the epithelial cells and is protected against proteolysis because it is released in combination with a transport piece.

IgD

IgD has no known protective role, and its function has yet to be determined. IgD has been found on the surface of a portion of cord blood lymphocytes in the neonate, and some investigators think that it may be an early receptor that later gives way to IgM and other immunoglobulins.

IgE

Only very low concentrations of IgE are present in the serum and only a few plasma cells are committed to its synthesis. It is known as the anaphylactic (reaginic) antibody and is responsible for the Type I hypersensitivity reactions. The contact of IgE with antigen results in the release of chemical mediators (e.g., histamine, serotonin, slow-reacting substance, bradykinin) from the mast cells. IgE antibody can remain fixed to mast cells for extended periods of time if injected into human skin. Serum levels of IgE are elevated in allergic states and parasitism. In parasitic infestation it is generally held that IgE bound to mast cells in the gut wall facilitates ejection of the parasite. IgE may also provide some natural defense mechanisms since patients who lack IgE have an increased susceptibility to respiratory infections. Some IgE is also found in secretions, i.e., tears.

Antigen Antibody Reactions

Reactions between antigens and antibodies take many forms. Precipitation, agglutination, opsonization, and complement fixation are the major forms of antigen antibody reactions.

Precipitation. Soluble antigens react with insoluble antibody complexes to form precipitates. These reactions are termed precipitation reactions.

Agglutination. Particulate antigens, such as red blood cells and bacteria, react with their homologous antibodies resulting in agglutinated aggregates.

Opsonization. Antibodies prepare bacterial surfaces to make it easier for the phagocyte to ingest. This process makes the bacterial wall "sticky," and these antibodies are called opsonins.

Complement Fixation. The humoral immunological response cannot be separated from another system called the complement system. The complement system serves as a nonspecific amplification of the HMI resulting in bacteriolytic reactions in which complement assists to lyse bacteria. It is a system present in serum which can be activated by antigen antibody reactions. The complement system's target is the antigen. When antigen is fixed to the cell membrane, the action of the complement system can result in irreversible damage to the cell. Complement is not thought to cross the placenta in humans. A number of researchers have found that neonatal titers of complement equal approximately half of the maternal titer. Based on these findings researchers believe that the complement system develops early in life and that it is independent of the B system.

Classical Pathway

The complement system can be activated by complexes of antigen and antibody or by discrete plasma proteins: C_1 (complex), C_2, C_3, C_4, C_5, C_6, C_7, C_8, C_9.

C_1 and its subunits bind in the presence of calcium to antibody. The C_1 bind C_4 and C_2, enhancing the phagocytic process. Next, C_3 is activated and directed into the reaction. Some fragments of C_3, which are chemotactic for polymorphonuclear leukocytes (PMN), are released. The combination of C_3 fragments and PMNs results in anaphylactic activity, e.g., histamine is released. C_3 on the cell surface causes the cell to be engulfed by white blood cells and hastens the formation of the next complement, complex C_5, C_6, and C_7, which attracts more white blood cells. C_8 and C_9 are

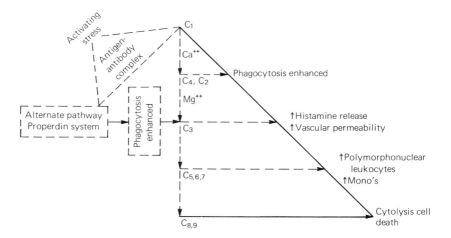

FIGURE 7   Complement system.

then activated and can physically damage the cell membrane. This interaction results in cytolysis. The C_1 complex appears to be located in the small intestine. C_2 may be made in large mononuclear cells of lymphoid tissues and peritoneal and lung exudates. C_3 and C_6 are probably found in the liver. Other sites involved in complement synthesis remain obscure. The activation of the entire complement system from C_1 and through C_9 is called the classical pathway or the complement cascade. The classical complement system may be better understood by reviewing Figure 7.

Alternate Pathway (Properdin Pathway)

Properdin, a distinct serum protein, is capable of activating C_3 in the absence of the C_1, C_4, C_2 complex, as well as in the absence of calcium. The complement complexes C_5, C_6, C_7, C_8, and C_9 act in the same order and manner seen in the classical pathway. The alternate pathway for activation of C_3 may be of importance in host resistance to extracellular bacterial pathogens and in neutralization of some viruses and some gram-negative bacteria. The alternate pathway spares the utilization of C_1, C_4, and C_2, and possibly functions as a host defense prior to antibody formation. This pathway is also depicted in Figure 7. Note that there is no difference between the pathways at the level of C_5, C_6, and C_7 activation.

SUGGESTED READINGS

Barrett JT: Basic Immunology and Its Medical Application. St. Louis, Mosby, 1976

Bigley NJ: Immunologic Fundamentals. Chicago, Yearbook, 1975

Cooper MD, Lawton A: The development of the immune system. Sci Am, 23:48–72, 1974

Good A, Fisher DW (eds): Immunobiology. Stanford, Conn, Senauer Associates Inc, 1971

Jerne SE: The immune system. Sci Am, 22:52–60, 1973

Maddison SE: Delayed hypersensitivity and cell mediated immunity. Clin Pediatr, 12:529–537, 1973

Nysather JO, Katz AE, Lenth JL: The immune system, its development and functions. Am J Nurs, October 1976

Roitt I: Essential Immunology. London, Blackwell, 1974

Stiehm RE, Fulginite VA: Immunological Disorders of Infants and Children. Philadelphia, Saunders, 1973

Turk JL: Immunology in Clinical Medicine. New York, Appleton, 1969

Weiser RS et al: Fundamentals of Immunology. Philadelphia, Lea and Febiger, 1970

CHAPTER THREE

Factors Differentiating the Humoral and Cell-Mediated Systems

As mentioned in a previous chapter, it has been through function rather than structure that we have come to understand the immunological system. In clinical practice it is important for nurses to understand the different means to evaluate humoral- and cell-mediated immunological (HMI and CMI) function. The rationale behind this evaluation comes from an understanding of the factors that differentiate humoral- and cell-mediated immunological function.

The foundation that determined these factors was laid in Chapter 2, where the structure and function of each system was discussed. This presentation is actually an analysis of that material and will compare and contrast concepts.

A careful analysis of the structure and function chapters provides the following areas that delineate the T and B cell function. These factors are source, development, life span, secretions, reactivity, specificity, tests of function, and clinical manifestations when deficiency is present. In addition, consideration should be given to T and B system interactions. Although this is not a differentiating factor, implications of this interaction are significant to the clinician in the assessment of either system and may provide the ability to predict possible outcomes.

TABLE 2 Source and Differentiating Influences of the T and B Systems

SOURCE	T	B	T AND B
	Stem cell	Stem cell	Stem cell
	Blood cells	Outer cortical regions of the	Loose connective tissue
	Yolk sac	lymph nodes	Efferent lymph channels
	Fetal liver		from regional nodes
	Bone marrow	Secretory medullary cords of the	Thoracic Duct
	Deep cortical areas of the lymph nodes	lymph nodes	Peripheral circulation
	Periarteriolar regions of the spleen	Red pulp of the spleen	
		Lamina propria region of the large and small bowel	
		Intestinal glands	
		Glands of external secretions	
Basis	Basis CMI	Basis HMI	
Cells	Small lymphocytes release lymphokines	Plasma cells release immunoglobulins	
Differentiating influence	Thymus	Genetic	Antigen stimulation

SOURCE AND DIFFERENTIATING INFLUENCE

Both T and B cells function as members of the lymphoid cell system. B cells (HMI) are developed from stem cells as are T cells (CMI). All have features of plasma cells and lymphocytes. B cells appear to develop from germinal centers in the outer cortical regions of the lymph nodes, the secretory medullary cords of lymph nodes, the *red pulp* of the spleen, the lamina propria regions of the large and small bowel, intestinal glands, and glands of external secretions. The differentiating influence appears to be genetically determined and stimulated antigenically. T cells are under the differentiating influence of the thymus gland; they develop from the blood cells in the yolk sac, fetal liver, and bone marrow, the deep cortical areas of the lymph nodes, and the periarteriolar regions of the spleen.

Both T and B cells are found in loose connective tissue, efferent lymph channels from regional nodes, thoracic duct lymph, and the peripheral circulation (Table 2).

DEVELOPMENT AND LIFE SPAN

T cells develop into the major component of the long-lived small lymphocyte population. Some have life spans of about 10 years. B cells can also be monitored over long periods of time. Each immunoglobulin secreted has a designated half-life and B cells maintain a capacity to secrete needed immunoglobulins when stimulated (memory) over periods of time.

SECRETIONS

T cells do not secrete immunoglobulins although some theorists propose that they are produced and held at the cell surface. They do produce several biologically active substances called lymphokines, which are able to kill nonspecifically, and engage in primitive reactive systems and biological amplification systems. Those identified include migration inhibition factor (MIF), lymphotoxic factor, skin-reactive factor, chemotactic factor, interferon, and antibody. B cells secrete immunoglobulins.

REACTIVITY

B cells respond to specific antigenic stimulation. The combination of the antigen with the antigenic receptor site occurs on the B cell surface and launches differentiation and proliferation of B cells. The reactivity mechanism for the T cell has not yet been determined.

SPECIFICITY

Specificity is at the cell surface of the circulating T lymphocyte. The antigen must come in contact with the T cell surface for a reaction to occur. B cells secrete immunoglobulins, and the antigen combining site is on the immunoglobulin molecule or point where the antigen engages with the amplification system.

ORGANISMS AND REACTIONS

T cells (CMI) are essential for life itself. They provide a readily mobile lymphoid pool that responds to invasion by fungi, viruses, facultative intracellular pathogens, and atypical acid fast organisms, such as Salmonella, Listeria, and Brucella. The mobilizable pool is responsible for delayed allergic reactions, the ability to reject solid tissue allografts, initiation of graft versus host reactions, and surveillance against malignancy.

B cells (HMI) provide major protection against high-grade encapsulate pyrogenic pathogens. They aid in the elimination of foreign red blood cells (RBC) and hematopoietic elements, assist with the elimination of certain viral infections, and can prevent stimulation by antigens that cross react with those of the host through local antibody systems.

COMBINED SELECTIVITY

The interaction of the T and B systems may be necessary for the maintenance of immunocompetency. Claman, in 1966, stated that B cells need to be present for appropriate and competent T cell immunodevelopment. In the B system, T cells also act to aid the antibody function of the B cells. The synergistic interaction between these systems is difficult to discuss because of the fact that judgment is based on clinical studies of hapten carrier conjugates. Haptens are small incomplete antigens which combine with high molecular weight carriers to incite antibody formation. The T

TABLE 3 T and B Systems: Organism Specificity, Functions, Tests for Functional Integrity, and Indicators of Dysfunction*

TESTS FOR FUNCTIONAL INTEGRITY

T-System
Organism specificity
 Fungi
 Virus
 Facultative intracellular
  pathogens
 Atypical host organisms
  (salmonella, listeria,
  brucella)
Functions

 Allergic reactions
 Rejection of tissue
  allograft
 Graft vs. host reaction
 In vitro response of cells
  to blast transformation
  and replication when
  stimulated with PHA
  phytohemagglutinin
  (allogenic cells)
Indicators of dysfunction
 Frequent viral infections
 Rubeola, rubella

 Renal failure
 Poor nutrition
 Alpha-globin factor

B-System
Organism specificity
 Polio virus
 Diphtheria-tetanus

 Polysaccharide antigens

Absence of defense against TB, fungi, virus,
 salmonella, SK-SD, mumps, candida, PPD
Contact allergy to 2,4 dinitrobenzene

Assesses population in deep cortical area of
 spleen; assesses capacity to reject allograft
MIF
Lymphocyte culture

Quantitative response to PHA
Dose response analysis to PHA response
Response of lymphocytes to allogenic, irradi-
 ated, or mitomycin-treated lymphocytes
Blood smear
Bone marrow aspiration

Complicated candida infections
Complicated rubeola, rubella, vaccinia
 infections
Proteus insufficiency

Antibody response to killed polio virus
Evaluate antibody response to polysaccharide
 antigens (pneumococcal, meningococcal,
 hemophilis)
(Table 3 Continued on p. 32)

*TB: Tuberculosis; SK-SD: Streptokinase Streptodornase; PPD: purified protein deriva-
tive; MIF: migratory inhibiting factor; PHA: physohemagglutinin; ASO: Antistrepto-
lysin titer.

TABLE 3 Continued

	TESTS FOR FUNCTIONAL INTEGRITY
Functions	
Secretions of immuno-globulins	Quantitative levels of major immunoglobulins
	Classes and subclasses (radioimmunoassay, radioimmunodiffusion)
	Evaluation of synthesis rates for individual immunoglobulins
	Evaluation of IgA content in saliva
	Evaluation of antibody concentrations in response to common antigens
	ASO titre
	Isohemagglutinins
Indicators of dysfunction	
Frequent infections: pneumococci, strepto-cocci, H influenza, meningitis, Pseudo-monas aeruginosa	Specific identification of causative organism
Viral hepatitis	Diagnosis of viral hepatitis
Sepsis, conjunctivitis	

cell is known to recognize the carrier molecule involved in triggering the formation of hapten-specific antibodies by B cells.

An understanding of the T and B systems' functions and differentiation has provided rationale for bone marrow transplants in combined immunodeficiency disease, as well as for thymic transplantation in the DiGeorge syndrome. Much has been derived from knowledge of the differentiation pathways of immunocompetent lymphocytes. There is still much to be learned regarding the events that precede induction and accompany the evolution of the specific immune response and its application to clinical problems. Individuals with intact B systems but defective T systems have unusual infections and are susceptible primarily to viruses and fungi. When the defect is in the B system, and the T system is intact, persons can handle most viruses well. Those with a T defect, but an intact B system, accept grafts without rejection. Those with a B defect and intact T system reject grafts. Table 3 summarizes the organism specificity and tests of function related to each system.

In conclusion, keep in mind that there is extreme danger from even small transfusions for those with T defects, because foreign allografts are not recognized as foreign. Therefore, transfused leukocytes react as if they were still in a normal environment, and host versus graft reactions occur.

SUGGESTED READINGS

Ackerman GA: Histochemical differentiation during neutrophil development and maturation. Ann NY Acad Sci 113:537–565, 1964

Bigley N: Immunological Fundamentals. Chicago, Yearbook, 1975

Burnet FM: Cellular Immunology. London, Cambridge Univ Press, 1969

Buxbaum JN: The biosynthesis, assembly and secretion of immunoglobulins. Semin Hematol 10:33, 1973

Claman HN, Chaperone EA, Triplett RF: Thymus-Marrow cell combinations —Synergism in antibody production. Proc Soc Exp Biol Med 122:1167, 1966

Cohn ZA: The structure and function of monocytes and macrophages. Adv Immun 9:163–214, 1968

David JR: Lymphocyte mediators of cellular hypersensitivity. New Engl J Med 288:143, 1973

Eldeman GM: The structure and function of antibodies. Sci Am 223:34, 1970

Good RA et al: Immunodeficiency diseases of man. In Amos B (ed): Progress in Immunology I. New York, Academic, 1971, p 699

Hong R et al: Hazards and potential benefits of blood-transfusion in immuno-deficiency. Lancet 1:1368–1369, 1964

Kirkpatrick CH et al: Chronic mucotaneous candidiasis: model building in cellular immunity. Ann Int Med 74:955–978, 1971

Lay WH, Nussenzweig V: Receptors for complement on leukocytes. J Exp Med 128:991–1007, 1968

Jerne NK: The natural selection theory of antibody formation. Proc Nat Acad Sci USA 41:849, 1955

Katz DH, Benacerraf B: The regulatory influence of activated T cells on B cell responses to antigen. Adv Immunol 15:1, 1972

Osgood EE: Regulations of cell proliferation. In Stohlman F (ed): The Kinetics of Cellular Proliferation. New York, Grune and Stratton, 1959

Reimer CB: Standardization of immunoglobulin reagents. Health Lab Sci 9:178, 1972

Roitt I: Essential Immunology. Oxford, Blackwell, 1971

South MA: IgA in neonatal immunity. Ann NY Acad Sci 176:40, 1971

Sprent J et al: Antigen-induced selective recruitment of circulating lympho-cytes. Cell Immunol 2:171–181, 1971

Sterzl J, Silverstein AM: Developmental aspects of immunity. Adv Immunol 6:337–459, 1967

Stiehm ER, Fulginiti VA: Immunological Disorders in Infants and Children. Philadelphia, Saunders, 1973

CHAPTER FOUR

Developmental Immunology

INTRAUTERINE CONCEPTS

The apparent harmony between the fetal-maternal unit remains an immunological enigma. Every fetus has paternal as well as maternal antigens and is thereby a potential allograft within the uterus. However, the fetus is immunologically protected from rejection, that is to say, it is exempted from immunological attack.

The lack of antigenicity in the fetus is attributed to the trophoblasts that secrete fibrinoid, creating an exempt site. So far, this hypothesis is the only acceptable one for the survival of the fetus in both normal and sensitized mothers.

Humoral System

The human fetus is capable of synthesizing its own immunoglobulins at an early age. Plasma cells are present but immunoglobulins are found only as traces, most likely due to the lack of antigenic stimulation. Immunoglobulins G and M are detectable in the fetus between 10 and 12 weeks. IgG is the only immunoglobulin known to cross the placenta, and it does so by a process that implies

35

active transport. Maternal-fetal transfer rates are dependent upon the IgG levels in the maternal-fetal circulation, as well as upon the age of the placenta. Low maternal levels result in low fetal levels.

IgM is the first immunoglobulin produced quantitatively by the fetus in response to primary antigenic stimulation. It would seem that IgM is the first line of defense against organisms entering via the bloodstream.

IgA makes an appearance about the 30th week. IgD has been found on the lymphocyte surface in cord blood and may be the precursor of IgM. The complement system develops early in intrauterine life and is independent of the production of immunoglobulin.

Cellular System

During intrauterine life the bone marrow cells come under the inductive influence of the thymus gland. Many cells are processed, but only a few leave the thymus, and these are called postthymic cells. The remainder of the developmental process is speculative. However, experiments do show that T cells constantly circulate in the lymphoid system, but do not return to the thymus.

The age at which the cell-mediated immune response (CMI) becomes competent in the fetus has not been determined. However, it is known that a premature infant is capable of rejecting transplants with a full immunological response. (CMI function has been detected as early as 12 weeks in fetal in vitro studies.)

CONCEPTS OF THE NEONATE

Humoral System

The neonate is partially protected during the first few weeks of life by passive maternal immunoglobulin G. However, maternal antibodies do have an immunosuppressive effect on the newborn, in that they delay newborn synthesis of IgG. As a result of normal catabolism of maternal IgG and a delay in newborn synthesis, there is a decrease in IgG levels in infants between two to six months (hypogammaglobinemia). This period is extended in the premature infant. Therefore, prematures are more vulnerable to neonatal infections. Postmature infants have higher levels of cord serum IgG and occasionally have elevated IgA. Infants with Down's syndrome have a decrease in maternal IgG levels. The presence of maternal IgG levels in the infant is the rationale used for delaying the initiation of immunizations until the second or third month of life. Maternal infections have a direct influence on neonatal infection, (e.g., premature rupture of the membranes, mycoplasma infections, etc.) and may result in low-birthweight infants.

IgM synthesis is accelerated in the newborn period. This is a result of the bacterial flora in the newly colonized gastrointestinal tract. IgM remains the predominant immunoglobulin synthesized by the newborn and is the one needed for protection against gram-negative organisms. Trace levels of immunoglobulins A, D, and E are present in the newborn's circulation.

In breast-fed infants colostrum supplies IgA as well as IgG. Secretory IgA is not absorbed, but will remain in the gastrointestinal tract. A few days after birth breast milk decreases in antibody content. It is possible that a breast fed baby may have more resistance to upper gastrointestinal infection than a bottle fed infant, because of the passive transfer of these immunoglobulins.

Complement is responsible for generating opsonization and chemotaxis. In the newborn there are decreased levels of complement. These levels correlate directly with birthweights. Also found are decreased levels of some of the alternate pathway components, e.g., properdin.

Infants are generally protected from infections due to pneumococci, H influenza, and meningococci. These are gram-positive organisms generally handled by IgG. Studies show that since 1954 gram-negative intestinal bacteria (*Pseudomonas aeruginosa, Proteus* species) are the leading causative agents of newborn septicemia. The use of penicillin could be responsible for this shift. Streptococcus group B is also among the leading etiological agents of neonatal sepsis.

Neonatal sepsis occurs more frequently in males than in females. The X chromosome controls the synthesis of immunoglobulins. Since the females carry two X chromosomes, they may have a higher heterogeneity to their antibody responses.

Colostrum supplies IgA as well as IgG. The longer the mother nurses, the more maternal IgG there is present. Secretory IgA is not absorbed but does remain in the gastrointestinal tract providing additional local protection against certain enteric pathogens.

Cellular System

The cellular system is harder to evaluate than the B system, which can easily be quantified in terms of antibody production. Skin tests were used initially in an attempt to measure T function. However, since there is a relative deficiency in phagocytic activity in the blood of infants, it could possibly inhibit the skin reaction. It has been proven that the neonate can reject an organ transplant, e.g., the thymus. The normal neonate has a structurally well-developed cell-mediated immune system.

   In summary, the structural components of phagocytic activity are present in the newborn. Qualitatively, the activity is still in a maturing process and is slow to function. Antigenic challenge is essential to the building of a complete, intense defense system for the human infant.

CONCEPTS OF THE NEONATE VERSUS THE ADULT

Intrinsic and Extrinsic Stress Factors

The neonate, when compared with the adult, is at a greatly increased risk when infected with a viral, bacterial, fungal, or protozoan organism. The bacterial infection rate in the neonatal group has remained the same over the past 30 years in spite of the use of antibiotics, and bacterial infections at this time in life are a major cause of death.

   Why is the picture so different in the adult, in whom the advent of antibiotics has provided a significant tool to combat infectious disease? Is the neonate more vulnerable to infection, or is the neonate inadequate in handling infections?

   Let us assess the internal and external stressors of the neonatal system. Conditions long known to be associated with extrinsically acquired infections in the neonate are premature rupture of the membranes, maternal infection, prolonged labor, contamination by equipment and/or personnel, and socioeconomic class.

However, the most important predisposing factor is an alteration in the neonatal immunological mechanism.

Alterations in the Neonatal Immunological Mechanism

The newborn, although competent in terms of having adequate numbers of T cells, does not respond in the same manner as the adult when exposed to an identical antigenic environment. The T cells in the newborn are not yet sensitized and thus have not become functionally competent.

Since the T cell promotes the production of substances that catalyze immunological responses, the infant, because of the lack of specificity in his T cell response, is at risk. Many neonatologists believe that, in spite of the fact that the newborn reacts to infectious antigens on a systemic level, he is unable to localize the response at the site of infection. In addition it has been noted that cord blood contains diminished numbers of T lymphocytes.

As mentioned earlier in this book, B cells produce antibodies in response to stimulation by antigen. They may act synergistically with T cells. B cell function in the newborn is also altered because of this synergistic effect. If the T cells respond slowly to antigenic stimulation, the B cells' production of antibody may also be reduced. Most newborns have not been exposed to infections in utero, and the antigen attraction of their B cells, which is present in the adult, may also be missing.

The human infant's B cell response appears to be intrinsically controlled. Even at term, newborns do not respond to a number of antigens. Inability to react adequately to certain antigens continues for the first 9 to 12 months of life. This is evidenced by the inadequate response to pneumococcal and H influenza capsules during the first 9 to 12 months of life.

The newborn is protected to a degree by his possession of maternal IgG transfused by the maternal-fetal-placental route. In addition the newborn exhibits an ability to produce IgM and IgG. IgG levels in the newborn correlate with the period of gestation and are equal or higher than maternal levels. It has, however, been documented that the preterm infant exhibits significantly lower levels of IgG.

It is possible that high levels of maternal IgG in the infant may reduce the ability of the newborn to respond to antigenic stimulation on its own, resulting in decreased levels of immunoglobulin at one year. Studies have indicated that the newborn develops antibody at a slower rate than the adult following immunization.

In the newborn decreased complement hemolytic activity and decreased complement components C_3, C_4, and C_5 have been found. Since the primary function of this system is to protect the organism from invading organisms through the generation of opsonic and chemotactic factors, it is not surprising that in the newborn the ability of the phagocytes in serum to ingest microorganisms is decreased. It is also of interest to note that the level of complement decreases as birthweight decreases.

Studies have also indicated that factor B and properdin are decreased in infants, possibly accounting for deficient opsonization capacties in the newborn. The decreased ability of newborn serum to produce chemotactic factors may be related to the newborn's inability to contain and localize microorganisms.

Lastly, consideration should be given to the functional capacity of the polymorphonuclear leukocytes (PMN) in the newborn. This is an area of controversy at present. It appears that PMN function does not correlate with birthweight, but possibly with preexisting stress.

Factors in neonates that appear to be altered when compared with older children and adults have been discussed in this chapter. It is believed that these factors act in conjunction with external stressors such as temperature, pathogens, air quality, etc., to precipitate infection in the newborn. The weighted importance of these factors, as well as the long-term developmental implications are questions yet to be investigated.

SUGGESTED READINGS

Alojipan LC, Andrews BF: Neonatal sepsis: a survey of eight years experience at The Louisville General Hospital. Clin Pediatr 14, 1975
Barr DCD: Infections. In Cockburn F, Drillen CM (eds): Neonatal Medicine. London, Blackwell, 1974, pp. 627–685

Buckley RH, Younger BJ, Brumley AW: Evaluation of serum immunoglobin concentrations in the perinatal period by use of a standardized method of measurement. J Pediatr 75(suppl):1143–1148, 1969

Davies PA: Bacterial infection in the fetus and newborn. Arch Dis Child 46: 1–27, 1971

Davis RH, Galontex SP: Nonimmune rosette formation: a measure of the newborn infants cellular immune response. J Pediatr 87:449–452, 1975

Fireman P, Luchowski DA, Taylar PM: Development of human complement system. J Immunol 103:25–31, 1969

Gotoff SP: Infections. In Behrman RE (ed): Neonatology: Disease of the Fetus and Infant. St. Louis, Mosby, 1973, p 129

Harris B: Neonatal-host defense mechanisms. Pediatr Ann 5:86–92, 1976

Host Defense Mechanisms in the Fetus and Newborn. Mead Johnson Symposium of Perinatal and Developmental Medicine. Evansville, Ind., November 27–29, 1972

Lawton AR, Cooper MD: Development of immunity: phlogeny and ontogeny. In Stiehm EH, Fulginiti VA (eds): Immunological Disorders in Infants and Children. Philadelphia, Saunders, 1973, p 33

Miller M: Chemotactic function in the human neonate: humoral and cellular aspects. Pediatr Res 5:487–492, 1971

McCrackin GH, Eichenwald HF: Leukocyte function and the development of opsonic and complement activity in the neonate. Am J Dis Child 121: 120–126, 1971

Rosen FS: Immunity in the fetus and newborn. In Gluck I (ed): Modern Perinatal Medicine. Chicago, Yearbook 1974, pp 273–283

Schaffer AJ, Avery MF: Diseases of the Newborn. Philadelphia, Saunders, 1971, p 632

Slansmith MR, McClellan BH, Butterworth M: Individual patterns of immunoglobulin development in ten infants. J Pediatr 75:1231–1244, 1969

Smith RT, Eitzman DVC: The development of the immune response: characterization of the response of the human infant and adult to immunization with Salmonella vaccines. Pediatrics 33:163–183, 1964

Stiehm ER: Fetal defense mechanism. Am J Dis Child 129:438–443, 1975

Stossel TR, Alper CA, Rosen FS: Opsonic activity in the newborn: role of properdin. Pediatrics 52:134–137, 1973

Washburn TC, Medeares DN, Childs B: Sex differences in susceptibility to infections. Pediatrics 35:57–64, 1965

Wilson HD, Eichenwald, HF: Sepsis neonatorum. Pediatr Clin North Am XXI:3:571–582, 1974

CHAPTER FIVE

Altered Immunocompetencies

Alterations in immunocompetency are primarily congenital and hereditary and, therefore, usually seen in infants and children. Most persons with alterations in immunocompetency exhibit an increased incidence of infections, especially at an early age of development. There are basically five types of immunocompetencies which relate to the structural categories of the immunological system: (1) immunoglobulin disorders (humoral, B cell), (2) cellular disorders (T cell), (3) combined defects, (4) complement disorders, and (5) disorders of phagocyte function. Alterations also occur as a result of illnesses that render the person temporarily or permanently susceptible to infections.

CLINICAL FINDINGS

The major symptom of immunoincompetency is the increased susceptibility to infection seen in these patients. There is an increase in the frequency of infections. Infections are more severe, unexpected and unexplained complications to infectious disease occur, common infections are present in an unusual manner, and infections occur as the result of exposure to an organism with low pathogenicity. Some findings usually consistent with hereditary immunoincompetency are recurrent respiratory infections, severe bacterial infections (such as pneumonia and meningitis), recurrent diarrhea, and failure to thrive. Clinical findings frequently present are draining ears, pallor and irritability, chronic pneumonitis or bronchiectasis, pyoderma, conjunctivitis, malabsorption, and inadeqaute development of the tonsils and lymph nodes. Thrush, vaccinia gangrenosa, skin rashes, severe viral disease, arthritis, hepatosplenomegaly, lymphadenopathy, and hematological disorders are occasionally present.

HISTORICAL FINDINGS

The history of patients with suspected immunoincompetency should be acquired in detail. A careful birth history should be included, noting maternal illnesses, length of gestation, birthweight, and a description of all neonatal illness. Immunization records are extremely important, since an adequate response to certain vaccines may indicate a competent immune system. The duration and quality of all cases of infectious disease are significant, because unusually severe cases of common childhood diseases are usually consistent with immunoincompetencies of varying degrees. The history as related to tolerance of formula and the addition of foods is also significant, as is the response to mechanical and chemical irritants. The nature of a rash, the manner of development, and the period of time the person exhibited the acute form may also give significant clues in the determination of immunoincompetency. Historical information should also include information related to tonsillectomy, adenoidectomy, radiation to the thymus or nasopharynx, and any prior gamma globulin therapy. Assessment of all medications given to the person and medications taken by the mother during pregnancy is also relevant.

The family history should include an investigation into the deaths of relatives, especially those of related children who died at an early age. Racial and national background, possible consanguinity, the presence of arthritis, collagen disease, allergy, and hypersensitivity in family members should also be evaluated.

PHYSICAL FINDINGS

Persons with immunoincompetencies usually appear chronically ill. They have pallor, inadequate subcutaneous fat, and distended abdomens. There are frequently abnormalities of the skin such as pyoderma, eczema, petechiae, alopecia, and macular skin rashes. There is frequently conjunctivitis of the eyes. The cervical lymph nodes are usually absent, in spite of frequent throat infections. The nasal turbinates are pink and difficult to visualize, and the nostrils are red and excoriated, with crusts present due to constant discharge. The tympanic membranes are scarred or perforated, and there may be discharge from the ear. Tonsils may appear to have been surgically removed. There are many adventitious chest sounds; rales are frequently heard; often there is hepatomegaly and splenomegaly. The presence of chronic diarrhea often leads to excoriation around the anal area. Joint motion may be limited, and there may be swelling of the joint. The presence of arthritis at times results in subcutaneous nodules. Development may be slow, neurological retardation evident, and ataxia sometimes seen.

LABORATORY FINDINGS

Tests for T and B System Competency

The initial laboratory work-up includes a blood count, a quantitative immunoglobulin analysis, a Schick test, an isohemagglutinin titer, and an evaluation of possible intrauterine infection (Torch test). In addition, a bone marrow biopsy may be performed. X-rays, antibody levels, metabolic studies, secretory antibody studies, and IgG subclass levels are also useful diagnostic tools. If cellular defects are suspected, then it is probable that other tests for cellular function will be performed after the initial work-up. X-rays can determine the presence of the thymus and can assess adenoidal tissue, which is usually absent in films of the lateral nasopharynx in persons with cellular immunoincompetency. Purified Protein Derivative (PPD) and Streptokinase–Streptodornase (SK–SD) tests are also of diagnostic value. Active sensitization with 2,4-dinitrochlorobenzene (DNCB) can also be used to assess cellular immunity.

In addition to the skin tests, the cellular immune system can be evaluated through determining the ability of the person's lymphocytes to proliferate and enlarge in vitro under the influence of an antigen. Observing the rate of rejection of a split thickness skin graft from an unrelated donor can also be of use in assessing delayed hypersensitivity, but it is rarely done. Morphological studies of biopsied lymph nodes also yield significant data. Lastly, assays for substances released by sensitized lymphocytes can be done.

Tests for Phagocytic Immunocompetency

Screening tests for phagocyte competency include a total leukocyte count, and differential and morphological evaluation. The presence of leukopenia or leukocytosis, or the presence of myelocytes in the peripheral blood is usually followed up by a bone marrow aspiration.

Scans are also done to evaluate the presence of the spleen. The Rebuck skin window is another test sometimes done to evaluate the morphology and function of cells in the inflammatory response. Another test done to assess phagocyte competency is the nitroblue tetrazolium test.

The simplest screening test for phagocyte competency is the slide test. In this test unstimulated leukocytes are mixed with nitroblue tetrazolium and incubated. The percentage of granulocytes containing formazan granules is then determined. The test evaluates metabolic activity of resting leukocytes. This test is useful to differentiate between viral and bacterial infections but cannot be used in newborns because they have high resting leukocyte metabolic activity. The tube test is another useful screening tool for leukocyte metabolic activity. A quantitative test of leukocyte metabolic activity was developed by Baehner and Nathan in 1967.

The most definitive test of function in the phagocyte is the quantitative bacterial phagocytic assay. This test measures phagocytosis and opsonic activity of serum and bactericidal activity separately. At times leukocytic bacterial iodination is utilized to assess the function of the leukocyte.

Tests for Complement and Opsonic Activity

These tests are utilized when patients with recurrent infections exhibit normal T and B cell function. First an evaluation of total serum complement is done. This is measured by radial diffusion. If this is abnormal, then complement component assays usually can be done. The tests available evaluate complement mediated function, assess phagocytic enhancement, chemotactic activity, immune adherence, and serum bactericidal activity.

The preceding discussion overviews the major historical, physical, and laboratory assessments used to evaluate the person with suspected immunoincompetency. Since many of the procedures are relatively new, they may not be available in all laboratories or treatment centers. In addition, research is producing new evaluation tools regularly. If a patient with immunoincompetency presents, the literature should be consulted to insure an adequate understanding of the screening and diagnostic evaluation.

IMMUNOINCOMPETENCY PROBLEMS ASSOCIATED WITH THE IMMUNOGLOBULINS

The immunoincompetencies of the immunoglobulin system are the following.

1. Immunoincompetencies of immaturity
2. Bruton's X-linked agammaglobulinemia
3. Normal or elevated IgG levels with an antibody deficiency
4. Acquired incompetencies
5. IgA deficiency
6. IgM elevation with decreased IgG and IgA

Immunoincompetencies of Immaturity

During normal development transient alterations of the immuno-globulin system occur. This is related to the passage of IgG anti-bodies from the mother to the infant. Neontal IgG levels are about equal to maternal levels, but only 20 percent of this IgG has been made by the infant. The maternal IgG passively protects the infant, but in addition suppresses active IgG synthesis. This is part of the reason that infants receive several diphtheria pertussis tetanus (DPT) and oral polio vaccine (OPV) immunizations, and why other vaccines such as measles and rubella are withheld until after one year of age. Usually by the end of the first year of life no significant residual amounts of maternal antibody remain to depress antibody production in the newborn. An assessment of IgM levels is of significant value. Elevated levels indicate the presence of intrauterine infection.

Intrauterine Infection

There are times when the infant does not begin to synthesize IgG until late. This may be due to residual amounts of maternal IgG, inadequate function of the B lymphocyte, or lack of adequate integration of the T and B systems. The result of this delay in ability to produce adequate immunoglobulin is infection in af-fected infants. At the age of 16 to 30 months, most infants are capable of producing adequate amounts of immunoglobulin. In the past, immunoglobulin therapy was utilized, but recent studies have indicated that this type of therapy can lead to delaying the development of the system even longer.

Bruton's X-Linked Agammaglobulinemia

Bruton's X-linked agammaglobulinemia is a sex-linked recessive immunoincompetency disorder; in fact, it was the first deficiency of immunoglobulins to be described. Children with this problem usually begin to exhibit increased susceptibility to infections after levels of maternal immunoglobulin dissipate. This occurs about the age of nine months. These children develop multiple and severe staphlococcal, streptococcal, pneumococcal, meningococcal, and hemophilus influenza infections. Although many viral infections provide no significant problems, secondary bacterial infection in chickenpox has been reported.

The lymph nodes in these patients appear to be absent upon palpation; x-ray findings illustrate the absence of the adenoids; isohemagglutinins are absent; and plasma cells are reduced in number when examination of the bone marrow is done. The clinical course of agammaglobulinemia has been altered since the development of more specific antibiotic therapy. However, repeated severe infections occur due to organisms that respond poorly to antibiotic therapy.

Because this is an X-linked recessive disorder, all of those affected are boys, and these children exhibit eczema, allergic rhinitis, rheumatoid arthritis, drug reactions, and autoimmune hemolytic anemia. Malabsorption syndrome is also seen, and these children are prone to disorders of the lymphoreticular system, such as lymphosarcoma. The therapy consists of gamma globulin administration. Prophylactic antibiotics are *not* recommended, but specific antibiotics should be utilized when sensitive pathogens are identified.

Immunoincompetency with Normal or Elevated IgG Levels

This is a poorly defined disorder in which immunoglobulin levels are normal or increased, yet the total antibody production response is poor with respect to specific organisms. Growth retardation, central nervous system symptoms, eczema, and glaucoma are frequently seen. Diagnosis is dependent upon identifying which antibodies are deficient. The cell-mediated system is functional, and therapy is usually dependent upon the administration of gamma globulin.

Acquired Immunoglobulin Incompetencies

These are conditions seen in both males and females and are not usually seen until after infancy. The disorders present with chronic or recurring infections complicated by eczema and rheumatoid arthritis. Prior to the onset of the disorders the immunological system is intact.

Defects of immunoglobulin production are seen in Hodgkins disease, lymphosarcoma, reticulum cell carcinoma, aplastic anemia, severe burns, exudative enteropathy, nephrotic syndrome, splenectomy, sarcoidosis, uremia, viral infections, and malnutrition.

Gamma globulin therapy may be utilized, but the response is temporary, and complications develop if the disorder is permanent. These complications present as autoimmune disorders, hemolytic anemias, neutropenia, and severe malabsorption syndromes.

Immunoglobulin System Incompetencies with Increased IgM Levels

In these disorders IgM levels are normal or elevated and IgG levels as well as secretory and serum IgA levels are absent. The onset of this condition is seen later than Bruton's agammaglobulinemia due to the fact that secretory IgM is the first immunoglobulin synthesized when a stressor presents and a temporary defense against invaders is available. This disorder appears to be a sex-linked inherited trait, but has also been attributed to intrauterine viral infections. The clinical findings are similar to those of children with Bruton's agammaglobulinemia but not as severe; thus the prognosis is similar and the treatment the same.

IgA Deficiency

The most frequently noted deficient immunoglobulin is IgA. IgA is both a serum component and a component in body secretions. Many times IgA is absent, and no clinical symptoms are present. Persons with chronic upper respiratory infections or chronic sinusitis at times are found to lack both types of IgA. Deficient IgA has also been associated with malabsorption syndromes. Of course, there are many persons with upper respiratory problems, sinusitis, and malabsorption problems who exhibit no alteration in IgA production.

There also appears to be a relationship between decreased IgA levels and disorders of autoimmunity. Although this is not always the case, the frequency of concurrence has supported the preceding hypothesis. The respiratory and gastrointestinal barriers are normally guarded by secretory IgA. When IgA is deficient, the absorption of protein and peptides normally excluded by functionally assistive secretory IgA may be permitted. These proteins may encourage the production of IgG and IgM antibodies. The cross reaction of these antibodies with related human molecules may result in a type of autoimmune reaction. Those autoimmune reactions that are frequently reported are rheumatoid arthritis and systemic lupus erythematosus. It has been reported that patients with IgA deficiencies have reacted with anaphylactoid shock following the administration of blood or plasma. Sarcoidosis, vascular and neurological disorders, and malignancy have also been reported.

There is no evidence that links IgA deficiencies to allergy or to IgE levels. The association of IgA deficit and genitourinary (GU) infections has been infrequently noted in the literature. There does appear to be a relationship between IgA deficiency and increased respiratory infections. Patients with malignancy or chromosomal abnormalities also appear to have decreased IgA levels.

There is also evidence to support the hypothesis that decreased IgA levels are associated with problems in the T cell system. This supports the concept of interaction between the two systems. The disorders where this phenomena is evident are ataxia-telangiectasia and eczema with thrombocytopenia. These problems will be discussed in the section on T cell system immunoincompetencies. Moderately depressed phagocytosis and chemotaxis is seen in children with Down's syndrome and is probably the reason behind the increased incidence of infection in these children.

Myeloperoxidase deficiency is a rare inherited disease which has associated diminished candidicidal activity but only mildly impaired bactericidal activity, suggesting that other pathways can compensate when any one is ineffective.

IMMUNOINCOMPETENCIES OF THE PHAGOCYTES

Polymorphonuclear leukocytes and mononuclear phagocytes both act to protect the human system against bacterial invasion. Their normal functions, as described in Chapter 1, protect the system by providing the mechanisms by which specific attachment, ingestion, and killing of bacteria occur, as well as by directing the movement of cells toward the site of stress. Genetic and acquired defects in any of these mechanisms result in the inability of the human immunological system to cope with stress due to bacterial invasion, and bacterial overgrowth occurs. Recent research has provided some insight into the significance of these defects, but future inquiry into more subtle defects will probably yield information of even greater consequence.

Genetic

Genetic defects of phagocytes cause alterations in bactericidal activity, chemotaxis, degranulation, locomotion, and candidicidal capacity. Some genetic defects of the phagocytes are discussed below.

Chronic granulomatous disease (CGD) is one of the genetically induced disorders of phagocyte function. The capacity of the phagocyte to kill gram-positive bacterial organisms as well as certain fungi is reduced. These organisms are known to cause severe and recurrent pneumonias, abscesses, and osteomyelitis, and children may exhibit severe recurrent pulmonary infections. Hydrogen peroxide and NADH (dihydronicotinamide adenine dinucleotide oxidase) production are also affected in chronic granulomatose disease.

CGD has two patterns of inheritance. In the typical pattern it is transmitted as an X-linked recessive trait. About 80 percent of those affected are males. The other pattern of transmission is via an autosomal recessive route. Females and a few males inherit the disease in this manner. CGD is frequently fatal in the first 10 years of life, but antibiotic therapy has assisted some patients to live into young adulthood.

Familial lipochromhistiocytosis is another genetically transmitted disorder of phagocyte function. Those affected are females and exhibit susceptibility to pulmonary disorders, rheumatoid arthritis, hypergammaglobulinemia, splenomegaly, and lipochrome pigmentation of histocytes. Bactericidal activity is diminished. The pattern of transmission is unknown, and the biochemical defect has yet to be defined.

Chédiak-Higashi syndrome, an autosomal recessive trait, has also been associated with disorders of phagocyte function. Job's syndrome presents with increased levels of IgE, depressed polymorphonuclear activity, and decreased chemotaxis. This syndrome has been reported only in females.

The "lazy leukocyte" syndrome is another disorder of phagocyte function. Persons with this syndrome exhibit stomatitis, gingivitis, otitis, and low-grade fevers but have normal T and B cell function. A peripheral neutropenia is present even though adequate numbers of mature polymorphonuclear leukocytes can be found in the bone marrow. The response of polymorphonuclear leukocytes to antigen antibody stimulation is depressed because of slowed random migration and decreased response to chemotactic factors.

There is evidence that suggests that the presence of ketoacidosis may impair other polymorphonuclear leukocyte (PMN) functions and account for the increased number of infections in children with poorly controlled diabetes.

Conditions such as candidiasis, systemic mycoses, and hypogammaglobulinemia also may be associated with chemotactic depression. Patients with advanced malignancy often exhibit depressed monocyte chemotaxis.

Certain pharmacological agents also affect phagocyte activity. Corticosteroids inhibit the bactericidal capacity of leukocytes. Sulfonamides, levorphanol (a morphine analogue), colchicine, and salicylates also have been reported to have a depressive effect on phagocyte function.

The future will probably provide additional evidence supporting the relationship of internal and external environmental conditions to altered phagocyte function. Nurses should be alert to such information as it provides the rationale for the institution of protective measures for those unable to deal with stressors as effectively as normal persons would. In other words, it will provide a rationale for health promotion during a period of risk.

Acquired

Often, one asks why one person exposed to an immunogenic stressor develops disease while another person exposed to a similar stressor stays healthy. This pattern is even more visible in the patient who has a chronic disease or who is vulnerable because of other environmental stressors. Conditions known to place a patient at risk are malnutrition, chemotherapy, radiation, infectious endocarditis, silicosis, severe burns, diabetes mellitus, ketoacidosis, and others. A stressor that has taken on additional significance in recent years is malnutrition. Evidence continues to accumulate that protein-calorie malnutrition as evidenced in children with kwashiorkor results in an increased incidence of infectious disease often leading to death. The phagocytic cells in these children function normally except for a decreased bactericidal activity and slowed chemotactic movement. Thus, increased susceptibility to bacterial infection results. Children receiving long-term hyperalimentation have also exhibited similar defects in phagocyte function.

Other populations at risk are children with disease such as myelogenous leukemia, in which function of phagocytes appears to be inhibited either by the disease or by chemotherapy.

Repeated spinal irradiation has also been associated with depressed phagocyte activity. Patients with infectious endocarditis exhibit diminished bactericidal activity toward staphylococcus aureus. Silica dust is toxic to alveolar macrophages, possibly accounting for the increased incidence of tuberculosis in persons with silicosis.

Severely burned patients exhibit defective neutrophil chemotaxis about a week after injury. This coincides with the bacterial invasion and sepsis noted at this time.

Patients with diabetes mellitus and severe bacterial infections have also been known to illustrate similar neutrophil defects.

IMMUNOINCOMPETENCIES OF THE T SYSTEM

A congenital disorder consisting of hypoplasia of the parathyroid glands, abnormal development of the third and fourth pharyngeal pouches, and thymic hypoplasia is known as the DiGeorge syndrome. The infant is born with abnormalities of the mouth and ears, and the eyes present with hypertelorism. There is a characteristic facies. Hypocalcemia is present, as well as histological abnormalities of the lymphocytes. The T system is not competent, yet the B system functions well. The immunoglobulin levels are normal.

The clinical picture consists of unusual susceptibility to infection in spite of adequate antibiotic therapy when indicated and normal immunoglobulin levels. Therapy consists of antibiotics known to be specific to the invading pathogen. Vitamin D and calcium supplements are provided because of the associated hypoparathyroidism. A low-phosphorus diet is usually recommended.

Thymic transplantation may be the recommended therapy. The transplant is frequently accepted by the donor even without histocompatibility typing, due to the fact that the cell-mediated immune response (CMI) is absent. If rejection occurs, the procedure must be repeated after compatibility typing has been done.

Those with limited hypoplasia have the best prognosis. Although providing a functional CMI is of importance, a copriority is to provide adequate therapy to prevent central nervous system damage resulting from hypocalcemic seizures.

Another disorder that alters the competency of the T cell system is chronic mucocutaneous candidiasis. The clinical picture consists of a severe persistent candida infection of the mucous membranes and skin. Diarrhea is also present in many affected infants. If diarrhea occurs, a massive candida infection of the diaper area results. Gastroenteropathy, swallowing difficulty, and granulomatous tissue changes result as the disease progresses. Most patients have an associated IgA deficiency as well.

Endocrinopathies (alterations in endocrine function) not associated with the candida infection often occur. Hypotheses exist associating this alteration in endocrine function to an autoimmune phenomenon. The endocrine alterations result in a host of additional symptoms related to the glands affected, such as diabetes mellitus, hypocalcemia, pigmentation, etc., due to idiopathic hypoparathyroidism and Addison's disease (adrenal insufficiency).

The classification of the endocrine problems is still controversial. Some researchers believe that it is a primary phenomenon, others feel that it is secondary to the initial defect.

This syndrome can present in the first days of life, infancy, adolescence, or in adulthood. A family history of candida is not uncommon. Treatment consists of providing antifungal agents to which the organism is sensitive. The use of topical preparations has not been of proven value. Intravenous amphotericin B has been used effectively as well as transfer factor isolated from the skin of subjects sensitive to candida. Amphotericin B is usually used prior to treatment with transfer factor. The treatment of the endocrine abnormalities is specific to the presenting endocrine problem, and is beyond the scope of this presentation.

COMBINED T AND B SYSTEM IMMUNOINCOMPETENCIES

Genetic

SWISS-TYPE AGAMMAGLOBULINEMIA

The most common and severe combined immunoincompetency disorder is what is usually called Swiss-type agammaglobulinemia. This is the most widely documented immunoincompetency disorder. Both the T and B systems are affected, there are no plasma or lymphoid cells, thymic dysplasia is present, and the histology of the lymph nodes is abnormal. The primary defect is in the stem cell itself.

Cases have been reported in males and females, but the disorder appears to be an X-linked recessive trait, thus three times more common in boys than girls. The clinical picture presents early in the neonatal period, even before maternal immunoglobulin stores have been depleted. Infection is the primary presenting symptom. Organisms creating problems for these children are of a broader group than those affecting children with Bruton's agammaglobulinemia. Organisms not usually considered pathogenic to man cause significant problems for these children. Those affected are prone to diarrhea, sepsis, skin infections, and bronchopneumonia. They are not protected against viral pathogens. Once maternal immunoglobulin stores are depleted, sepsis occurs and is severe if not fatal.

Thymic transplant has been attempted unsuccessfully in the past. However, histocompatible bone marrow transplants have been used recently and are believed to provide a degree of immunological competence.

IMMUNOINCOMPETENCY OF NEZELOF

Nezelof has described another type of immunoincompetency that is a combined T and B cell defect. It is a recessive autosomal trait, lymphopenia occurs, and IgG production is altered. The thymus is dysplastic, and plasma cells appear normal. The alteration in the IgG appears to be an alteration in the specificity of antibody production. Investigators hypothesize that their defect is a developmental defect of the bone marrow stem cell and of the genes that control the synthesis of the IgG molecule.

The clinical picture consists of symptoms that present in late infancy or early childhood. They are quite similar to the symptoms reported for other types of combined immunoincompetency, except for a relatively normal IgG level and the late age of onset. The thymus is abnormal as are the lymph nodes. There are fewer than 2000 lymphocytes per cubic millimeter. Although IgG levels are normal, this does not correlate with the antibody response. Patients suffer from severe viral and mycotic infections that are frequently fatal. Again, bone marrow transplants have been used more successfully than thymic transplants.

RETICULAR DYSGENESIS

Another type of congenital disorder is reticular dysgenesis. The bone marrow precursors, as well as the cells of the T and B systems, are affected. The clinical picture consists of vomiting and diarrhea, sepsis, and failure to thrive. Patients have normal hemoglobin and platelets. The illness is quite severe, and death occurs before six months of age. One hopes that earlier diagnosis will permit histocompatible bone marrow transplant in the future.

COMBINED IMMUNOINCOMPETENCY
WITH ATAXIA TELANGIECTASIA

An autosomal recessive disorder consisting of immunoincompetency with ataxia telangiectasia presents with progressive cerebellar disease, multiple ocular and cutaneous telangiectatic sites (small flattened dilated or raised vascular nodules which blanch with pressure), and combined immunodeficiency. IgA production is usually affected, as well as the thymus and the T system. They may also exhibit a deficiency of IgE. Telangiectasia of the central nervous system occurs, as well as gonadal defects. There are two possibilities in regard to the primary defect. Either there is a defect in embryogenesis, or an autoimmune phenomenon develops subsequent to the thymic dysplasia, causing damage to other organs. At present there appears to be no hypothesis to explain the multiple sites affected.

The clinical picture consists of ataxia as the infant begins to walk. The disability is progressive. Choreoathetoid movements, facial and eye movements which appear to be tics, and cerebellar abnormalities are present. The picture of recurrent infections is consistent with IgA immunoincompetencies. However, the frequency and severity is increased due to the deficiency of the T system. As mentioned earlier, the two systems act together and facilitate each other in terms of providing a defense against invaders. There is also clinical evidence to support the fact that malignancy and autoimmunological problems are more frequent in these patients.

The prognosis is varied; some patients have lived up to 40 years, others succumb early to the disease process. There is a relationship between the severity of the disease and treatment potential: The more severe the disease, the less effective the treatment. Gamma globulin therapy has not been effective. A transient beneficial effect from plasma transfusions has been reported. This effect lasts from three to four weeks. If radiation therapy is required for patients with malignancy, the possibility of infection increases because radiation therapy has a suppressive effect on an already less than competent immunological system.

WISKOTT-ALDRICH SYNDROME

The Wiskott-Aldrich syndrome is a sex-linked recessive disorder of the immunological system. There is a combined defect of the immunological system, and eczema and thrombocytopenia are present. The disease involving the immunoglobulin system is progressive resulting in decreased IgM production and the variable production of IgG. There is an increase in IgA and IgE synthesis. There is a progressive development clinical process manifested by symptoms of increasing severity related to the production of immunoglobulins.

The child usually presents with thrombocytopenia and petechiae. There is a characteristic atopic dermatitis (eczematoid rash) that appears about the age of six months. An excessive number of severe infections occur as the child grows older. Studies have shown that the infections are due to viruses and nonbacterial organisms. The child does not have allergies except for the eczema. The frequency and severity of the infections increase with age. Since the disorder initially presents with bleeding problems, the diagnosis of the combined immunoincompetency is often delayed, especially in the first affected male. Tests of both limbs of the immunological system are conclusive by the sixth month of life. Since this is a progressive disorder, the number of competent thymic cells decreases with age. As in most disorders to the immunological system, there are histological abnormalities of the lymph nodes.

Treatment is dependent on management of the bleeding disorder and control of the immune defect. Steroid therapy is used to alleviate the thrombocytopenia as well as to manage the eczema. The use of steroids often masks the early signs of infection and thus allows the progression of the infectious process. This provides a most serious side effect in patients with this disorder, as bacterial infections must be identified early and specific therapy instituted. Splenectomy, once used in the treatment of thrombocytopenia, has recently been noted to increase the severity of the problem. Nursing observations both of environmental variables and signs of early infection become highly significant to the management of patients treated with steroids.

The use of transfer factor isolated from lymphocytes of normal subjects has been somewhat effective in the treatment of this combined disorder of the immunological system. The number of infections has been reduced as well as the number of cases of atopic dermatitis. Thrombocytopenia is, however, not improved. This therapy must be repeated about every six months. The most ideal therapy proposed would be the transplantation of histocompatible bone marrow.

Bleeding episodes in major organs or hemorrhaging elsewhere seem to determine the prognosis of this disorder in the younger child. As the child becomes older, the probability of severe infection increases and acts as a survival determinant. In addition, as the child becomes older, he is more susceptible to lymphoreticular malignancies that introduce a host of additional problems in terms of therapy.

ADENOSINE DEAMINASE DEFICIENCY

A disorder resulting from the lack of essential enzyme called adenosine deaminase presents in almost exactly the same way as the combined form of immunoincompetency, except for the fact that the disorder is primary and due to the absence of the enzyme. The enzyme is absent in multiple tissues. Abnormalities of the spine, pelvis, and ribs are seen in about one-half of these patients. This is an autosomal recessive trait, and if suspected can be diagnosed before birth by amniocentesis. The treatment is similar to that used for other types of immunoincompetency disorders of the combined type. Histocompatible bone marrow transplants are used, and the transplantation of fetal liver plus thymus has been shown to be somewhat effective.

SHORT-LIMBED DWARFISM WITH IMMUNOINCOMPETENCY

A recessive autosomal disorder that presents with short-limbed dwarfism as well as immunoincompetency is another type of combined immunoincompetency problem. There is no evidence to explain why the short-limbed dwarfism occurs. There is also a hypoplasia of the cartilage and hair. There seems to be a sex-linked determinant to the inheritance of these features. The joints are loose, but the extension of the elbow is limited. There is a defect in the sternum. Due to the associated features the diagnosis is usually made at birth, and the treatment for the immunoincompetency is similar to that utilized for the other types of immunoincompetency.

THYMIC TUMOR WITH ASSOCIATED COMBINED
IMMUNODEFICIENCY

A combined immunoincompetency disorder is associated with thymic tumor, and both benign and malignant tumors have been associated with this disorder. A relationship between bone marrow abnormalities and thymic abnormalities is known and it is hypothesized that an autoimmune phenomenon is involved. Treatment is aimed at the specific symptoms manifest in the individual patient, as mentioned in relationship to the other types of immunoincompetency that have been discussed. Gamma globulin injections have been of some use. Tumors of the thymus should be removed. This will not affect the immunological problems, but the hematological problems should improve.

Acquired

Acquired immunoincompetencies result in the loss of a previously effective immunological system. There is a developmental perspective to this problem, as it often occurs in old age. There is also an association between acquired immunodeficiency and malnutrition. The nutritional basis appears to be hypoproteinemia. This type of hypoproteinemia may result from nephrotic syndrome or from a malabsorption syndrome. The malabsorption problems develop as a result of the gluten malabsorption syndrome in those with food and milk sensitivity and in intestinal lymphangiectasia. Other syndromes that may have an associated protein loss are constrictive pericarditis, cystic lymphangiomas, Whipple's disease, chronic ulcerative colitis, and regional enteritis.

The clinical picture consists of recurrent respiratory infections, Candida skin infections, bone marrow hypoplasia, and thrombocytopenia involving the stem cells. The lymph node histology is altered as in other types of immunoincompetency. The thymus and IgA-containing plasma cells appear normal. The treatment is similar to that utilized for other types of immunoincompetency problems and is directed at the presenting system of deficit.

IMMUNOINCOMPETENCIES RESULTING FROM ALTERATIONS IN THE COMPLEMENT SYSTEM

Immunoincompetencies related to disorders of the complement system involve both the components of the system itself, as well as specific inhibitors that regulate the components of the system.

Most relate to genetic alterations and affect the human organism's resistance to invading pathogens as well as to the disease process itself.

The normal function of the complement system was described in Chapter 3. Since that chapter relates specifically to normal function, it may be useful to refer to this material if confusion develops relative to a specific disorder. Almost all disorders discussed are currently under study and controversial in many respects.

C_1 Deficiency

Hereditary angioneurotic edema is an hereditary deficiency of C_1 esterase inhibitor. It is hypothesized that this is an autosomal dominant trait. Massive edema occurs in affected persons as a result of absent or defective inhibition. In essence, the C_1 molecule is overactive. Complement components C_2 and C_4 are present in lower levels than seen in normals.

C_2 Deficiency

Patients with lupus erythematosus at times manifest C_2 deficiencies. It was once thought that C_2 disorders were associated with few clinical symptoms, but research is changing this perspective. There is much study in progress regarding C_2 deficiency. Patients with C_2 deficiencies may exhibit a variety of collagen vascular-like syndromes.

C_3 Deficiency

C_3 deficiency has been reported, but research and clinical evidence regarding this entity are limited. All patients have exhibited recurrent bacterial infections, and it appears that a deficiency of C_3 activity can result in clinical abnormalities. Alper has reported a hereditary condition in which C_3 levels are about 50 percent of what is expected in normals. A deficient inhibitor to C_{3b} has been identified. This results in excessive stimulation of the (properdin) alternate pathway, which is also deficient when C_3 is deficient. The clinical picture again consists of recurrent infections.

C_4, C_5, C_6, C_8 Deficiencies

C_4 deficiency has been associated with systemic lupus erythematosus. C_5 deficiency has also been reported. In these cases C_5 levels were normal, but the molecules exhibited abnormal opsonic and chemotactic activity. Function was altered, and therefore recurrent infections resulted. C_6 deficiency has recently been reported in humans. This condition has been extensively studied in rabbits, where there is an associated defect in the blood clotting mechanism. Further investigation regarding this condition in humans may yield significant data regarding the inflammation process. C_8 deficiency was identified in a patient with a protracted case of severe gonococcal sepsis. C_6 and C_8 have been found in patients with gonococcemia whose serum lacked bactericidal activity.

Alternate Pathway

Alterations in the C_1 and C_3 components do not appear to produce marked clinical symptoms. This is related to the presence of the alternate pathway (properdin pathway) and to the degree of acceptable variation in complement component levels before clinical manifestations present. Complement function and dysfunction are open areas for research at this time, and future research will probably change our present perspective considerably.

CONCLUSION

At this point in time it is sufficient to state that complement is significant to health in man. A determination of normal complement ranges has recently been proposed and should provide a useful adjunct to further investigations regarding complement activity. The determination of total complement levels is now available in many centers; however, it will be some time before a complement component assay is a feasible diagnostic tool. These tests are available in only a few laboratories and are extremely complicated and expensive.

SUGGESTED READINGS

Immunoincompetency Problems
Associated with the Immunoglobulins
Ament ME: Immunodeficiency syndromes and gastrointestinal disease. Pediatr Clin North Am 22:807, 1975
Ammann AJ, Hong R: Ataxia-telangiectasia and autoimmunity. J Pediatr 821, 1971
Ammann AJ, Hong R: Selective IgA deficiency: presentation of 30 cases and a review of the literature. Medicine 50:223, 1971
Ammann AJ, Roth J, Hong R: Recurrent sinopulmonary infections, mental retardation and combined IgA and IgE deficiency. J Pediatr 77:802, 1970
Bellanti JA, Schlegel RJ: The diagnosis of immune deficiency diseases. Pediatr Clin North Am 18:49, 1971
Bruton OC: Agammaglobulinemia. Pediatrics 9:722, 1952
Buckley RH, Wray BB, Belmaker EZ: Extreme hyperimmunoglobulinemia E and undue susceptibility to infection. Pediatrics 49:59, 1972
Cassidy JT, Norby GL: Human serum immunoglobulin concentrations: prevalence of immunoglobulin deficiencies. J Allergy Clin Immunol 55:35, 1975
Cassidy JT et al: Selective IgA deficiency in connective tissue disease. N Engl J Med, 280:275, 1968
Conn HO, Quintillani R: Severe diarrhea controlled by gamma globulin in a patient with agammaglobulinemia, amyloidosis, and thymoma. Ann Intern Med 56:528, 1966
Crabbe PA, Heremans JF: Selective IgA deficiency with steatorrhea: a new syndrome. Amer J Med 42:319, 1967
Douglas SD, Goldberg LS, Fudenberg HH: Clinical, serological and leukocyte function studies on patients with idiopathic "acquired" agammaglobulinemia and their families. Amer J Med 48, 1970
Evans DIK, Hotzel A: Immune deficiency state in a girl with eczema and low serum IgM. Arch Dis Child 54:527, 1970
Feingold M et al: IgA deficiency associated with partial deletion of chromosome 18. Amer J Dis Child 117:129, 1969
Gatti RA et al: Hereditary lymphopenic agammaglobulinemia associated with a form of short limbed dwarfism and ectodermal dysplasia. J Pediatr 75:675, 1969
Hitzig WH et al: Heterogeneity of phenotypic expression in a family with

Swiss type agammaglobulinemia: observations on the acquisition of agammaglobulinemia. J Pediatr 78:968, 1971

Lai a Fat RFM, McClelland DBL, Van Furth R: In vitro synthesis of immunoglobulins, secretory component, complement, and lysozyme by human gastrointestinal tissues. I. Normal Tissues. Clin Exp Immunol 23:9, 1976

Miller WV et al: Anaphylactic reactions to IgA: a difficult transfusion problem. Am J Clin Pathol 54:618, 1970

Polmar SH et al: Immunoglobulin E in immunodeficiency diseases. I. Relation of IgE and IgA to respiratory tract disease in isolated IgE deficiency, IgA deficiency and ataxia telangiectasia. J Clin Invest 51:326, 1972

Radi J, Masopust J, Lacova E: Selective hyperimmunoglobulinemia A and D in a case with chronic generalized eczema and prolonged sepsis. Helv Petriatr Acta 22:278, 1967

Stiehm ER, Fulginiti VA: Immunological disorders in infant and children. Philadelphia, Saunders, 1973

Vyas GN et al: Serologic specificity of human anti-IgA and its significance in transfusion. Blood 34:573, 1969

Waldmann TA, Strober W, Blaeses RM: Immunodeficient disease and malignancy: various immunological deficiencies of man and the role of the immune processes in the control of malignant disease. Ann Inter Med 77:605, 1972

Waldmann TA et al: Thyoma, hypogammaglobulinemia and absence of eosinophils. J Clin Invest 46:1127, 1967

Immunoincompetencies of the Phagocytes

Craddock PR et al: Acquired phagocyte dysfunction: A complication of parenteral hyperalimentation. New Engl J Med 290:1403, 1974

Daughaday C, Douglas S: Phagocytes. Pediatr Ann 5:18, 1975

Davis SD, Schaller J, Wedgwood R: Job's syndrome. Lancet 1:1403, 1966

Douglas SD: Disorders of phagocyte function: analytical review. Blood 35:85, 1970

Douglas SD, Schoffer K: Phagocyte function in protein calorie malnutrition. Clin Exp Immunol 17:121, 1974

Hill HR, Quie PG: Raised serum IgG level and defective neutrophil chemotaxis in three children with eczema and reoccurrent bacterial infection. Lancet 1:183, 1974

Marsh WL, Uretsky SC, Douglas SD: Antigens of the kell blood group system on neutrophils and monocytes: their relation to chronic granulomatous disease. J Pediatr 87:1117, 1975

Miller ME, Oski FAC, Harris MD: Lazy-leukocyte syndrome: a new disorder of neutrophil function. Lancet 1:665, 1975

Immunoincompetencies of the T System

Buckley RH et al: Defective cellular immunity associated with chronic mucocutaneous moniliasis and recurrent staphylococcal botryomycosis: immunological reconstitution by allogenic bone marrow. Clin Exp Immunol 3:153, 1968

Cahill LT, Ainbender E, Glade PR: Chronic mucocutaneous candidiasis: T cell deficiency associated with B cell dysfunction in Man. Cell Immunol 14:215, 1974

Chilgren RA et al: The cellular immune defect in chronic mucocutaneous candidiasis. Lancet 1:1286, 1969

DiGeorge AM: Congenital absence of the thymus and its immunological consequences: concurrence with congenital hypoparathyroidism. In Bergsma D, Good RA, (eds): Immunological Deficiency Diseases in Man (Birth Defects 4:1). Baltimore, Williams and Wilkins, 1968

Gajl-Peczalska KJ et al: B and T lymphocytes in primary immunodeficiency disease in man. J Clin Invest 52:919, 1973

Gatti RA et al: DiGeorge syndrome associated with combined immunodeficiency. J Pediatr 81:920, 1972

Giblett ER et al: Nucleocide-phosphorylase deficiency in a child with severely defective T cell immunity and normal B cell immunity. Lancet 1:1010, 1975

Kappe S et al: Variable cell-mediated immune defects in a family with "Candida endocrinopathy syndrome." Clin Exp Immunol 20:397, 1975

Lischner HW: DiGeorge syndromes. J Pediatr 81:1042, 1972

Salvin SB, Peterson RDA, Good RA: The role of the thymus in resistance to infection and andotoxin toxicity. J Lab Clin Med 65:1004, 1965

Say B et al: Thymic dysplasia associated with dyschondroplasia in an infant. Am J Dis Child 123:240, 1972

Stiehm ER, Fulginiti VA: Immunological Disorders in Infants and Children. Philadelphia, Saunders, 1973

Wanderer AA, Go S, Ellis EF: Late-onset hypogammaglobulinemia with cellular immune deficiency. J Pediatr 78:278, 1970

Combined T and B System Immunoincompetencies

Ackeret C, Pluss HJ, Hitzig WH: Hereditary severe combined immunodeficiency and adenosine deaminase deficiency. Pediatr Res 10:67, 1976

Bach FH et al: Bone marrow transplantation in a patient with the Wiskott-Aldrich syndrome. Lancet 2:1364, 1968

Bellanti JA, Schlegel RJ: The diagnosis of immune deficiency diseases. Pediatr Clin N Amer 18:49, 1971

Bensel RW, Stadlan EM, Krivit W: The development of malignancy in the cause of the Aldrich syndrome. J Pediatr 68:761, 1966

Biggar WD, Good RA, Park BH: Immunoreconstitution of a patient with combined immunodeficiency disease. J Pediatr 81:301, 1972

Conn HO, Quintiliani R: Severe diarrhea controlled by gamma globulin in a patient with agammaglobulinemia, amyloidosis, and thymoma. Ann Int Med 56:528, 1966

DiGeorge AM: Congenital absence of the thymus and its immunological consequence: concurrence with congenital hypoparathyroidism. In Bergsma D, Good RA (eds): Immunological Deficiency Disease in Man (Birth Defects 41). Baltimore, Williams and Wilkins, 1968

Douglas SD, Fudenberg HH: Graft vs host reaction in Wiskott-Aldrich syndrome ante mortem diagnosis of human GVH in an immunologic deficiency disease. Vox Sang 16:172, 1969

Gatti RA et al: Hereditary lymphpenic agammaglobinemia associated with a distinctive form of short-limbed dwarfism and ectodermal dysplasia. J Pediatr 75:675, 1969

Hermans PE et al: Dysgammaglobulinemia associated with nodular lymphoid hyperplasia of the small intestine. Am J Med 40:78, 1966

McKusic AV, Cross HE: Ataxia telangiectasia and Swiss-type agammaglobulinemia. Two genetic disorders of the immune mechanism in related Amish sibships. JAMA 195:739, 1966

McKusic AV et al: Dwarfism in the Amish. II. Cartilage-hair-hyperplasia. Bull Johns Hopkins Hosp 116:285, 1964

Meuwissen HJ, Pollara B, Pickering RJ: Combined immunodeficiency disease associated with adenosine deaminase deficiency. J Pediatr 86:169, 1975

Nelson DL et al: Constrictive pericarditis, intestinal lymphangiectasia, and reversible immunological deficiency. J Pediatr 86:548, 1975

Parkman R et al: Severe combined immunodeficiency and adenosine deaminase deficiency. N Engl J Med 292:714, 1975

Root AW, Speicher CE: The triad of thrombacytopenia, eczema, and reoccurrent infection (Wiskott-Aldrich syndrome) associated with milk antibodies, giant cell pneumonia and cytomegalic inclusion disease. Pediatrics 31:444, 1963

Say B et al: Thymic dysplasia associated with dyschondroplasia in an infant. Am J Dis Child 123:240, 1972

Wanderer AA, Go S, Ellis EF: Late-onset hypogammaglobulinemia with cellular immune deficiency. J Pediatr 78:278, 1971

Immunoincompetencies Resulting from
Alterations in the Complement System

Agnello VM, deBracco ME, Kunkel HG: Hereditary C_2 deficiency with some manifestations of systemic lupus erythematosus. J Immunol 108:837, 1972

Alper CA, Rosen FS: Genetic aspects of the complement system. Adv Immunol 14:251, 1971

Alper CA et al: Homozygous deficiency of C_3 in a patient with repeated infections. Lancet 2:1179, 1972

———, Studies in vivo and in vitro on an abnormality in the metabolism of C_3 in a patient with increased susceptibility to infection. J Clin Invest 49:1975, 1970

Ballow M et al: Complete absence of the third component of complement in man. J Clin Invest 56:703, 1975

Day NK et al: C_2 deficiency: development of lupus erythematosus. J Clin Invest 52:1601, 1973

Donaldson VH, Evans RR: A biochemical abnormality in hereditary angioneurotic edema. Am J Med 35:37, 1963

Hauptman GE, Grosshans E, Heid E: Systemic lupus erythematosus and hereditary complement deficiencies: a case with total C_4 deficiency. Dermatol Syphilige, 101:479, 1974

Klemperer MR et al: Hereditary deficiency of the second component of complement (C_2) in man. J Clin Invest 45:880, 1966

Leddy JP et al: Hereditary deficiency of the sixth component of complement in man. 1: Immunochemical, biologic and family studies. J Clin Invest 53:544, 1974

Miller ME et al: A familial plasma-associated defect or phagocytosis: a new cause of recurrent bacterial infections. Lancet 2:60, 1968

Muller-Eberhard HJ: The molecular basis of the biological activities of complement. Harvey Lect 66:75, 1972

Norman ME et al: Serum complement profiles in infants and children. J Pediatr 87:912, 1975

Peterson BH, Graham JA, Brooks, GF: Human deficiency of the eighth component of complement. J Clin Invest 57:283, 1976

CHAPTER SIX

Conditions that Alter the Immune Response

FACTORS INFLUENCING
THE EFFECT OF IMMUNOLOGICAL STRESS

The human system is in contact with and inhabited by microorganisms, some of which are necessary for normal function. This normal flora is generally considered nonpathogenic. However, there are times when the functional capacity of the host-defense system is compromised, and infection results. Infection as a result of invasion by a microorganism that does not generally produce disease in a normal healthy person is termed opportunistic infection. These infections could and should be anticipated and diagnosed early. Appropriate medical and nursing therapy should then be instituted as soon as possible. It should be emphasized that problems altering the host defenses confer the potential of pathogenicity to the microorganism involved.

At greatest risk are patients with chronic debilitating disease. These patients are subject to long hospitalizations, intravenous infusions, and a host of additional factors that make them more vulnerable to invasion by microorganisms. Other factors influencing host–defense activity are endocrinopathies, renal failure, sickle cell anemia, asplenia, malnutrition, cystic fibrosis, malignancy, and organ transplants. The following material is a discussion of these factors and the related host response under the stress of primary disease.

ASPLENIA SECONDARY
TO SICKLE CELL ANEMIA

Children with homozygous sickle anemia are compromised hosts. They exhibit increased susceptibility to infectious stressors. Their diminished defenses may be the result of inadequate function of the liver and spleen. The spleen and reticuloendothelial systems are ineffective as a filter for microorganisms, because they are involved in the trapping of abnormal red blood cells. There is also an unexplained decrease in opsonic activity (one of the steps in the process by which antigens are prepared for destruction). Thus, the white blood cell has a more difficult time destroying the antigen.

Those affected exhibit increased susceptibility to Diplococcus pneumonia, *Hemophilus influenzae,* Salmonella, and Mycoplasma. The most common sites of infection are the lungs, bones, meninges, and genitourinary tract. Persons with functional asplenia (absence of spleen function), other than sickle-cell disease, who are at risk following a splenectomy are those with thalassemia, Hodgkins' disease, Wiskott-Aldrich syndrome, histiocytosis, lipidosis, and portal hypertension.

CYSTIC FIBROSIS

Cystic fibrosis (CF) is an autosomal recessive genetic disorder of the exocrine glands. It affects many organs, predominantly the pancreas and the lungs. There are pancreatic enzymes, such as tripsin, lipase, and amylase, that are absent or available in limited quantities. The mechanism responsible for monitoring the concentration and composition of exocrine secretions is altered in some manner. These patients are stressed with repeated infections.

Innate cilia and mucous mechanisms which normally screen and protect the respiratory tract against bacterial invasion are defective. The mucoid secretions are viscid, resulting in obstruction of the bronchial lumina and stasis. The viscid mucous decreases motility and further stasis results. This stasis of the mucoid secretions provides an excellent medium for bacterial growth. Early colonization with *Staphylococcus aureus* and *Hemophilus influenzae* results, because the normal mechanisms for clearing debris from the respiratory tract are ineffective.

Frequently children develop resistant organisms, especially *Pseudomonas aeruginosa,* which are associated with an increased mortality rate. Intensive antibiotic therapy is used in recurrent progressive disease.

It has been noted that serum levels of immunoglobulin are elevated in these patients. IgA is elevated in saliva and serum. IgG levels are very high and reflect repeated antigenic stimulation. Rule has found IgA in the meconium of cystic fibrosis infants. This led to a clinical application of Rule's findings. A screening test for CF with an immunological basis was developed in 1968 by Grunard Schwachman. In this test antisera to human protein is utilized to detect the presence of undigested serum proteins in meconium.

UREMIA WITH NEPHROTIC SYNDROME: RENAL FAILURE

Immunological activity and response in patients with uremia is depicted by a variety of abnormalities, such as increased susceptibility to infection and an altered response to organ transplants. Uremia causes varying degrees of immunological anergy (reduced ability to function).

In spite of antibiotics, there is still a high incidence of pneumococcal peritonitis in nephrotic syndrome patients. Enteric induced infection is now on the increase in these patients. Those patients on steroid and/or cyclophosphamine therapy may develop severe infections secondary to measles or varicella.

Lymphopenia is a frequent occurrence. There is a depressed delayed hypersensitivity reaction to Purified Protein Derivative (PPD) and histoplasmin, mumps, Candida, and coccidioidin. The presence of these inadequate delayed hypersensitivity reactions is probably related to a depression of T cell function. This is also evidenced by an increased incidence of infection by *Pneumocystis carinii,* herpes virus, and fungi.

Humoral function as well as neutrophil activity appears normal. There is research in progress on the effects of this syndrome on the early phases of the inflammatory response. Alterations associated with this response are suspected.

MALNUTRITION

The interrelationship between malnutrition and infection has been the subject of much research. Scrimshaw has studied this area extensively. He demonstrated that there are two immunological activities resulting from this interrelationship. One is synergistic and cooperative, while the other is antagonistic and inhibiting. Generally, synergism increases the frequency of infections, while antagonism decreases the frequency of infections or limits their severity.

In malnutrition, synergism results and provides an optimal environment for bacterial infections, rickettsial infections, and helminth infestations. Protozoal infections are also increased. The incidence of viral infections is less in those with malnutrition when compared to the normal population. Protein deficiencies result in synergism for infection as do deficiencies in vitamins A and C. Deficiencies of vitamin B and several minerals result in both antagonistic and synergistic activities, depending on the host and organisms. There is also a decrease in reticuloendothelial activity, which affects antibody production and phagocytosis.

The state of nutrition or the type of malnutrition are relevant to the duration and severity of the infections involved. Protein-calorie malnourished children show growth retardation, dermatitis, apathy, peculiar moon faces, abnormal hair, and splenomegaly. Cholesterol and serum proteins are decreased as well as gastrointestinal enzymes, such as lipase, amylase, and esterase. The children are frequently anemic.

Infections are recurrent with pneumonia being the most common. The most serious infections are those due to gram-negative organisms in the gastrointestinal and genitourinary tracts and in the blood. Salmonella is often isolated from these areas. Measles, even without the rash, can be fatal and are often complicated by giant cell pneumonia. Infestation with parasites is common. Herpes viral infections are high in morbidity during malnutrition.

It appears that there may be some impairment in the primary antigen-antibody response in persons with severe protein-calorie malnutrition. The competency of hemolytic complement activity is also questioned and is an area requiring further investigation. Cellular lymphopenia is also present in 25 percent of children with protein-calorie malnutrition. There is evidence suggesting a lack of delayed hypersensitivity reactions in those affected. Thymic atrophy, depleted peripheral lymphoid tissue, and paracortical cells are also present. These findings are seen in malnutrition and other chronic debilitating diseases.

Depressed T function may account for the number of parasitic infestations in those with protein-calorie malnutrition. Investigators have attempted to use transfer factor from parents to treat these children. This has resulted in a decreased number of infections.

TRANSPLANTS

Organ transplant recipients on immunosuppression therapy are more prone to infection and more vulnerable to malignant diseases. Some of the drugs used to suppress the immune response are steroids, cyclophosphamine, purine analogs, and methotrexate. Another extrinsic therapeutic mechanism used to suppress the immune response are large doses of irradiation. Both chemotherapy and radiotherapy depress the bone marrow and the functions of the immunological system. Although these therapies are vital to transplant acceptance, they do leave the recipient increasingly more vulnerable to infection from opportunistic organisms and/or multiple infective agents.

Among the significant data now available it has been noted that the incidence of verrucae is increased in transplant recipients if there was a history of childhood warts. This may be related to a reactivation of a latent virus. About 90 percent of transplant patients exhibit cytomegalovirus. It has been suggested by some investigators that this virus may be activated by allogenic reactions (allograft rejections). The transplantation and rejection process itself may alter the host defenses, and predispose the patient to infection.

ENDOCRINOPATHY

Knowledge of the effects of endocrine influences on leukopoiesis is limited and largely descriptive. Patients with overproduction of adrenal steroids show erythrocytosis, neutrophilia, lymphopenia, and eosinopenia. Underproduction of adrenal steroids results in anemia, neutropenia, lymphocytosis, and eosinophilia. In the diabetic patient, leukocytes exhibit decreased chemotactic activity. When glucose levels are high, there appears to be a decrease in leukocyte phagocytic function. An increase in blood sugar slows the inflammatory response due to sluggish polymorphonuclear response and lack of fibroblast proliferation. This results in ineffective phagocytosis. Metabolic acidosis also contributes to this problem.

In patients with diabetes mellitus the absorption of intramuscular injections may be delayed or inhibited, resulting in a reduced effect of antibiotic therapy. Infections due to *Staphylococcus aureus, Escherichia coli, Proteus,* Clostridia, and Actinomyces frequently are seen in diabetics as well as perinephric abscesses and pyelonephritis. The use of antibiotics has resulted in an increase in Candida and mucormycosis fungal infections in these patients.

MALIGNANCY

There has been a high incidence of infection associated with patients who have some form of cancer. Obstruction and invasion may enhance infection by causing abnormalities in local host defenses.

The potential for infection development depends on the form of cancer and its treatment. Generally, lymphopenia occurs and predisposes affected patients to fungal and viral infections. Delayed hypersensitivity, anergy, as well as impaired macrophage function have been noted in some patients with malignancies. They are increasingly more susceptible to salmonella, brucella, listeria, tuberculosis, some fungi, and intracellular organisms. There is an increased incidence of fatal *Pneumocystis carinii* infections in children with acute leukemia who are receiving chemotherapy.

Surgery, irradiation, and chemotherapy used to treat patients with malignancies provide rich environments for infective agents. There are many intrusive measures used, such as needles, catheters, and respirators. These are all additional portals of entry for infectious agents. Any one of these measures increases the probability of infection, but when used together the effect is synergistic and probabilities become realities. Complications of therapy, such as mucosal ulcers, poor wound healing, and malnutrition also support the growth of microorganisms.

One organism, *Pneumocystis carinii,* occurs almost exclusively in conditions where immunosuppression is present, e.g., cancer patients, debilitated patients, protein-calorie malnutrition patients, and transplant recipients. This organism is rarely pathogenic in healthy individuals.

SUGGESTED READINGS

Asplenia Secondary to Sickle Cell Anemia

Barrett-Connor E: Bacterial infection and sickle-cell anemia. An analysis of 250 infections in 166 patients and a review of literature. Medicine 50: 97–112, 1972

Diaz F, Mosovich LL, Neter E: Serogroups of Pseudomonas aeruginosa and the immune response of patients with cystic fibrosis. J Infect Dis 121: 269–274, 1970

Eraklis AJ et al: Hazards of overwhelming infection after splenectomy in childhood. N Engl J Med 276:1225, 1967

Pearson HA, Spencer RP, Corneliers FA: Functional asplenia in sickle-cell anemia. New Engl J Med 281:923, 1969

Saslow S et al: Studies on antibody response in splenectomized persons. N Engl J Med 261:120, 1959

Shulman ST, Bartlett J, Clyde WA Jr, Ayoug EM: The unusual severity of mycoplasmal pneumonia in children with sickle-cell disease. N Engl J Med 287:164–167, 1972

Robinson MG, Watson RJ: Pneumonoccal meningitis in sickle-cell anemia. N Engl J Med 274:1006–1008, 1966

Cystic Fibrosis

Beggir WD, Holmes B, Good RA: Opsonic defect in patients with cystic fibrosis of the pancreas. Proc Natl Acad Sci USA 68:16–17, 1971

Cahill LT: Impairness of natural defenses. II. Endogenous causes. Pediatr Ann 5:457–464, 1976

Green MN, Kulczycki LL, Schwackman H: Serum protein paper electrophoresis in patients with cystic fibrosis. Amer J Dis Chil 100:365–372, 1960

Green MN, Schwackman H: Presumptive tests for cystic fibrosis based on serum protein in meconium. Pediatrics 41:989–992, 1968

Gugler C, Pallavicini JC, Swerdlow H, Zipkin L, di Sant'Agnese PA: Immunological studies of submaxillary saliva from patients with cystic fibrosis and from normal children. J Pediatr 73:548–559, 1968

Halbeck SP, di Sant'Agnese PA, Koter FR: Staphylococcal antibodies in cystic fibrosis of the pancreas. Pediatrics 26:792–799, 1960

Rule AH, Baron DT: Quantitative determination of water soluble proteins in meconium. Pediatrics 45:847, 1970

Stiehm E, Fulginiti VA: Immunological Disorders in Infants or Children. Philadelphia, Saunders, 1973

Uremia with Nephrotic Syndrome: Renal Failure

Long PA, Ritzmann SE, Merian FL, et al: Cellular evolution in induced inflammation in uremia patients. Texas Rep Biol Med 24:107–111, 1966

Riott I: Essentials of Immunology. London, Blackwell, 1974

Tescban PE: On the pathogenesis of uremia. Am J Med 48:671–677, 1970

Wilson WEC, Kirkpatrick CH, Talmage DW: Suppression of immunologic responsiveness in uremia. Ann Intern Med 62:1–14, 1965

Malnutrition

Formos ML, Stiehm ER: Impaired opsonic activity and normal phagocytosis in low birth weight infants. N Engl J Med 281:926–931, 1969

Jose DG, Ford GW, Welch JS: Therapy with parents lymphocyte transfer factor in children with infection and malnutrition. Lancet 1:263, 1975

Klainer AS, Beisel WR: Opportunistic infections: a review. Am J Med Sci 258:431, 1968

Reddy V, Srikantia SG: Antibody response in kwashiorkor. Indian J Med Res 52:1154–1158, 1964

Scrimshaw NS, Taylor CE, Gordon JE: Interactions of nutrition and infection. Am J Med Sci 237:367, 1959

Stiehm E, Fulgineti V: Immunologic Disorders in Infants and Children. Philadelphia, Saunders, 1973

Weiser RE, Myrvik QN, Pearsall NH: Fundamentals of Immunology. Philadelphia, Lea and Febiger, 1970

Transplants

Barnett JT: Basic Immunology & Its Medical Application. St. Louis, Mosby, 1976

Butt K, Kountz SL: Transplantation immunology. Association of Operating Room Nurses Journal 20:589-599, 1974

Cahiel L: Impairment of natural defense. II. Endogenous courses. Pediatr Ann 5:457-464, 1976

Leonard M: Nephrology nursing: interplay of skills. Association of Operating Room Nurses 20:597-601, 1974

Weller TH: The cytomegaloviruses. Ubiquitous agents with protean clinical manifestations. N Engl J Med 285:203, 1971

Malignancy

Armstrong D et al: Infectious complications of neoplastic disease. Med Clin N Am 55:3, 1971

Gooch WM, Femback DJ: Immunoglobulins during the course of acute leukemia in children. Effects of various clinical factors. Cancer 28:984, 1971

Hughes WT et al: Intensity of immunosuppression therapy and the incidence of pneumocystis carinii pneumonitis. Cancer 36:2004, 1975

Hughes WT, Feldmen S, Cox E: Infectious diseases in children with cancer. Pediatr Clin N Am 21:583, 1974

Wilbur JR et al: Chemotherapy of Sarcomas. Cancer 36:765, 1975

CHAPTER SEVEN

Physiological Reactions Mediated by the Immune System: Allergy

IMMUNOLOGICAL INJURY

Allergy is a form of immunological injury. It is a reaction or alteration mediated by the immunological system which can be detrimental to the human system. Originally, allergic phenomenon were categorized according to four types of reactions. These categories were described by Gell and Coombs, and Roitt has added a fifth classification. The reaction types are as follows: Type I, anaphylactic; Type II, cytotoxic; Type III, immune complex mediated; and Type IV, cell-mediated injury. The fifth type proposed is antibody-mediated stimulation injury.

These types of reactions and their clinical significance are described in the first section of this chapter. The second section considers a type of immunological injury in which there is a loss of the immunological ability to tolerate self antigens. This phenomenon is known as the autoimmune response. The third and last section of this chapter deals with another form of immunological injury which is proposed to be due in part to the loss of ability to recognize what is indeed a foreign antigen, the tumor cell. This third section deals with a discussion of the surveillance role of the immunological system. Theories describing altered mechanisms in

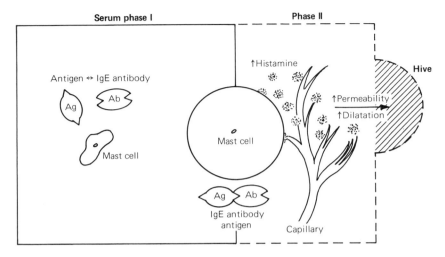

FIGURE 8 IgE-mediated anaphylactic reaction: the reaction of antigen with IgE antibody results in fixation of the antigen and antibody on the mast cell. The mast cell degranulates releasing pharmacologically active material. The resulting tissue changes, either local or systemic, are caused by these pharmacological agents.

relationship to the development and limitation of malignancy will also be discussed.

The chapter as a whole should provide an in-depth understanding of the structures involved and the functions of the immunological system in allergy. A prospectus regarding the effect of these reactions on the total human system and the role of nursing practice in this area is also included.

TYPES OF ALLERGIC REACTIONS

Type I: Anaphylactic Reaction

This type of reaction is best known as the immediate hypersensitivity reaction. It is mediated in most cases by IgE, but several reports indicate that IgG can also act as a mediator. Individuals with IgE-mediated hypersensitivity reactions develop allergies after sensitization with ingested, injected, or inhaled antigens. The mechanism responsible for this reaction is described in Figure 8.

In phase I (immune reaction), a specific antibody is formed in the serum in response to antigenic exposure. In phase II (allergic reaction), the antibodies that have been released into the blood become attached to mast cells in the tissues. The subsequent exposure of the system to a similar antigen causes an interaction between the antibodies attached to the mast cell wall and the antigen. This results in destruction of the mast cell. During this process the mast cell deposits granules containing histamine or mediator substances (slow-reacting substance [SRS], other chemotactic factor, and other vasoactive factors). Calcium ions and enzymes act upon these granules, which mediate the release of histamine into the intercellular spaces. There the histamine acts at receptor sites and may produce eczema, rhinitis, congestion, tearing, smooth muscle spasm or systemic vasodepression. This reaction occurs within seconds to minutes following exposure in sensitive individuals. An extensive anaphylactic reaction can lead to respiratory failure and death.

The immediate reaction consists of a wheal and flare inflammatory reaction (a hive). There is pruritis and the site may be painful. Wheals develop wherever the antigen that has produced the allergic state interacts with cell-bound IgE in the interstitial tissue. Those reactions resulting from food allergies develop after the ingested antigen has been digested. The allergenic substances are then released into the circulation.

These responses may be local or systemic. The next section will consider some of the common reactions found in a normal population and consider pertinent nursing implications.

INGESTED ANTIGENS

Food Allergies. Clinical problems associated with food allergies are seen most frequently during the first few years of life. This is probably related to the fact that following this period the sensitive individual has developed an awareness of the antigens that cause allergic reactions and is able to avoid them. At present there is no easy laboratory method available to detect food allergy. The elimination diet is the most useful diagnostic tool. Once an offending food is identified it is eliminated from the diet. The use of injection therapy has not been effective in the management of food allergies.

There is a broad role for the nurse practitioner in the management of the patient with food allergies. The diet history is of great significance, and nurses can assist in acquiring discriminating data in this area. Family history is also of significance and is often accurately related only after the development of meaningful interpersonal relationships. The nurse should provide time for this type of interaction to occur. The elimination of offending foods from the diet may prove difficult from the points of view of both nutritional management and economics. In collaboration with the physician and dietitian the nurse can assist the family in planning meals that are personally and culturally acceptable, as well as economically feasible. Last but not least, a great deal of support, reassurance, and education is required for successful management of the problem.

Drug Allergies. Allergies to drugs may result in skin reaction if the medication is a topical preparation, a gastrointestinal reaction if the medication is given orally, or a systemic response if the medication is given parenterally. Even limited contact can result in a systemic response if the individual is sensitized.

Drug-induced skin reactions. There has always been controversy in categorizing skin reactions. This is partially due to the fact that there is an endless variety of skin reactions that can occur. It is thought that some of the long-acting sulfonamides are associated with the development of Stevens-Johnson syndrome, but it is difficult to explain why in other patients receiving these preparations erythemia nodosum occurs. It has been suggested that the primary disease for which the preparation is given may have some effect on the resulting reaction. There have been rashes reported during ampicillin therapy, which seem to occur more frequently in patients whose response is altered by glandular fever.

Contact dermatitis may result from medications or from chemical agents. These are sometimes treated as antigens and combine with the tissue proteins in the epidermis. Either the IgE-mediated hypersensitivity-type reaction or a delayed-type hypersensitivity reaction may occur (Type IV). The treatment of this type of problem is removal of the offending antigen and avoidance of this preparation in the future.

There has been little written about *intestinal allergy* and medications. However, there have been cases reported in which vomiting and diarrhea occur immediately after the administration of a specific preparation. The identification of appropriate antibodies has not yet been determined, but there appears to be a relationship between this reaction and Type I allergy.

INJECTED ANTIGENS

Insect Bites and Stings. The order Hymenoptera is almost entirely responsible for the insect bites and stings from the class insecta which result in hypersensitivity reactions. This order includes ants, bees, hornets, and yellow jackets. The clinical picture manifested by the reaction may vary from a generalized urticaria, angioedema, itching, anxiety, wheezing, respiratory difficulty, cyanosis, dysphagia, abdominal pain, dizziness, confusion, circulatory collapse, to evidence of anaphylaxis. This type of generalized reaction assumes a previous sensitizing sting. Delayed responses have been reported and may occur within 24 hours to 10 days following the bite or sting. These reactions produce a serum sickness-like syndrome consisting of fever, joint pain, and urticaria. The manifestations of a delayed-type reaction may occur with the initial sting. It appears that there are antibodies other than IgE which are capable of mediating this response, or that the reaction to some insect stings is not an immunological hypersensitivity reaction. This statement is based on attempts made to correlate skin test reactions with sensitivity states. There is no consistent correlation between levels of circulating antibody and clinical sensitivity.

It is usually difficult to determine the exact type of insect that caused the bite or sting. Studies have revealed that much information related by subjects following the sting is unreliable. Even though one type of insect caused the initial hypersensitivity, the patient could be sensitive to more than one of the Hymenoptera. Cross sensitivity is not uncommon, and all of this group should be used for testing and treatment.

A systemic allergic response is usually easily determined by historical and physical evidence. The person taking the history should be careful not to overlook other possibilities that could account for similar symptoms. Immediate hypersensitivity reactions have been categorized into four graded areas. In a Grade I reaction there is generalized urticaria, itching, malaise, and anxiety. A Grade II reaction consists of any of the Grade I symptoms plus two or more of the following: generalized edema, constriction in the chest, wheezing, abdominal pain, nausea, vomiting, dizziness. A Grade III reaction is a severe general reaction and consists of any of the symptoms exhibited in a Grade II reaction plus two or more of the following: dyspnea, dysphagia, hoarseness or thickened speech, confusion, feeling of impending disaster. The Grade IV reaction is a shock reaction and consists of any of the symptoms in a Grade III reaction plus the addition of two or more of the following: decrease in blood pressure, cyanosis, vascular collapse, incontinence, unconsciousness.

The treatment of acute reactions consists of the administration of epinephrine. This should be given promptly in a dose that will protect the patient against total anaphylaxis. Antihistamines and steroids are sometimes used to control lingering urticaria, angioedema, or other anaphylactic symptoms. Aerosol epinephrine has been used to effectively treat respiratory distress. If self administration is necessary, isoproterenol is given by a sublingual route. Isoproterenol has been of value in providing time until the patient can receive medical attention, however, isoproterenol will not prevent respiratory failure. Any person given this preparation should be aware that further therapy may be required to prevent death. Steroid therapy does not seem to be of value in the treatment of an immediate hypersensitivity reaction, in that the preparation does not act quickly enough and time is one of the most important variables in the treatment of these patients.

The degree of the reaction almost always increases following the initial sensitization. It is not possible to predict if the reaction to subsequent exposure will reach fatal consequences. It is on this basis that most clinicians recommend prophylactic treatment for all persons having a systemic reaction of any degree to an insect bite or sting. This treatment should be in the form of specific hyposensitization injection therapy. Local reactions to bites and stings do not require immunological treatment. However, recent studies have indicated that those who developed increasingly severe localized reactions later had a high incidence of severe generalized reactions. The presence of positive skin tests in these patients indicates the development of a systemic response and are an indication for hyposensitization therapy.

The patient should not be scheduled for skin testing until at least two weeks following the acute systemic reaction. Patients may be in a refractory period at this time and have little or no antibodies available to react. This will result in a false-negative reaction.

Immunological treatment consists of the administration of whole body extract of bee, wasp, hornet, and yellow jacket. It has been reported to provide protection in 70 to 95 percent of cases. The initial dosage is usually equal to the amount of dilution that resulted in a positive skin test. Increasing doses are then administered on a regular schedule until a maintenance dose level is achieved. The antigenic component of the maintenance dose is equal to the antigen dose received after two to four stings. The time period of immunization varies, but many clinicians recommend that therapy be carried on at monthly intervals for one year after the maintenance level is achieved, at bimonthly intervals for the second year, and at three month intervals for the third year, and then discontinued. This procedure is of course dependent on the individual allergist. A booster dose on an annual basis has been suggested to insure protection.

There is no distinct guidelines related to the time required for desensitization. However, a period of about two to three years of uninterrupted therapy is recommended by the Insect Allergy Committee of the American Academy of Allergy.

The patient is advised that protection cannot be expected for at least two years and in some cases three years. Protective measures recommended prior to desensitization include the following:

1. Avoid Hymenoptera stings
2. Carry an emergency kit at all times

The likelihood of incurring a sting can be decreased by

1. Not wearing colognes and perfumes
2. Not walking barefoot through grass, especially clover
3. Not wearing bright-colored garments
4. Carrying and using a deterrent insect spray or cream if in proximity to insects

Patient education should be provided related to the emergency kit. Most contain epinephrine in a sterile syringe, antihistamine, and tourniquet. These kits are available commercially or can be improvised at home by purchasing the components at the pharmacy. Immediately following a sting, the patient should inject epinephrine, and apply a tourniquet if possible above the level of the sting. The application of a cold compress is helpful. The antihistamine should be taken following the injection of the epinephrine. Upon completion of first-aid procedure, professional assistance should be sought from the nearest clinic, hospital, or physician.

The treatment of patients with this type of hypersensitivity reaction should be under the close supervision of a physician who has had experience with this form of therapy, as well as with the life-threatening consequences of an anaphylactic reaction. In addition, nurses working with this type of patient have a responsibility to continually update their knowledge in this area, as there are frequently times when they must make crucial decisions. The community health nurse should also be familiar with the therapeutic principles related to this area of practice, as it is not uncommon for parents and/or family members to seek advice regarding problems in this area. Actually, all nurses should have a strong working knowledge of concepts related to immediate hypersensitivity reactions should their immediate intervention become necessary. Table 4 is a quick reference chart showing what one sees and does when an insect bites. Health education for all health care consumers should include content related to the management of Type I hypersensitivity reactions due to injected types of antigens.

INHALED ANTIGENS

Many persons are allergic to airborn substances such as dust, pollen, mold, and animal dander. The respiratory tract is the region most commonly affected by Type I allergic reactions. These allergic disorders commonly give rise to allergic rhinitis (hay fever) and asthma. There is frequently a familiar tendency toward this type of reaction.

Hay fever is a good example of a local allergic hypersensitivity reaction. This disorder affects the upper respiratory tract and conjunctiva. Pollens react with cell-bound immunoglobulin E, and mediator substances are produced which cause the release of histamine. This causes vasodilation and increased capillary permeability, with a resulting edema in the surrounding tissues and an increase in secretions. If the response is limited to the upper respiratory tract, the response is a profuse rhinorrhea. Hypersecretion, bronchospasm, and edema signal lower respiratory tract involvement and may signal respiratory obstruction and an asthmatic attack. In many cases it has not been possible to identify the offending allergen, but skin testing has provided the identification of the responsible allergens in some cases that were formerly thought to be of vasomotor origin.

This clinical picture depicts the allergic response that is seen in relationship to most respiratory antigens. There is a predictable local response that can become systemic and result in an asthmatic attack. Many patients with respiratory allergies are treated with medications. This is a necessary therapy and at times it is life saving. However, there is also a need to find and eliminate the cause of the symptoms. If the cause is identified and removed the symptoms will disappear.

The treatment utilized currently for asthma consists of avoidance, hyposensitization, cromolynsodium, and symptomatic care. The avoidance of causative factors is the most important concept. The better the avoidance the smaller the amount of medication needed. The better and more complete the avoidance, the more likely hyposensitization therapy will be effective. If avoidance is adequate and proper hyposensitization therapy utilized, fewer and fewer drugs will be required. Lastly, the occurrence of status asthmaticus and death from asthma would decrease.

Although the administration of medication and manipulation of fluid and electrolyte balance, blood gases, and dilution factors is of great significance, time and energy spent preventing severe allergic asthmatic episodes is also very important and there is a feasible nursing role in this latter effort.

Household Allergens. The house dust antigen develops from the breakdown of animal and vegetable matter present in upholstered furniture, carpet pads, and drapes. In recent years, the house dust mite has been postulated to be the house dust antigen, especially by the Dutch. However, American investigators have illustrated through skin testing and inhalation testing that there are many

TABLE 4　A Quick Reference to Insect and Spider Bites and Stings

WHAT IS SEEN	WHAT TO DO
Insects	
Normal Reactions	
Small red area at sting site in minutes	Do not pull out stinger.
Hive formation	Scrape external debris away with finger nail.
Itching	If bite has occurred in the eye or other delicate area, surgical removal is required.
Disappears in a few hours	Clean area with soap and water.
	Ice packs may reduce swelling and discomfort.
Toxic reactions may be due to multiple stings	Do not use heat.
GI symptoms, edema, headache, fever, muscle spasms, drowsiness, convulsions	Seek medical help if hives occur.
Infected Reactions	Seek medical help at once.
Cellulitis	Clean site. Analgesics for pain.
May be gas gangrene	Oral sedatives.
Can occur hours to days after stings	IV fluids, antibiotics, and antihistamines may be required. Observe carefully.
Generalized Reactions	Seek medical assistance.
Occur in minutes	Systemic antibiotic therapy may be required.
Dry hacking cough	
Dyspnea	**Now:** Seek medical assistance at once.
Asthma, cyanosis, abdominal cramps, diarrhea, nausea, vomiting, chills, fever, vertigo, stridor, shock, unconsciousness, incontinence	Subcutaneous　IM aqueous epinephrine 1:100, 0.3cc-0.5cc for adults, 0.2-0.3cc for children. Massage injection site.
	Observe closely. Vital signs 5-15 min/1 hr.
	Aminophylline IV is required if the condition does not improve.

Adapted from Frazier, C.A. "A Guide to Insect Bites and Stings" Pediatric Basics 15: 14-15, 1976.

TABLE 4 Continued

WHAT IS SEEN	WHAT TO DO
	Intramuscular antihistamine is usually injected after the epinephrine.
	Steroids in IV drips may prolong the effects of epinephrine and antihistamine.
	O_2 will minimize hypoxia.
	B/P and circulatory support measures may be required.
	Cardiovascular collapse can occur.
	Plasma expanders are sometimes used to ensure adequate blood volume and cardiac output.
	Later: Give insect sting kit, educate regarding use.
	Provide with medic alert bracelet which identifies their allergy to insect stings.
	Use avoidance measures until hyposensitization from therapy complete.
	Advise to start hyposensitization.
Delayed Reactions Fever, malaise, headache, urticaria, polyarthritis 10–14 days following sting.	Dependent on symptoms. See "Generalized Reactions."
Spiders* *Black Widow* Subject may be unaware he has been bitten. Sharp pin prick sensation, numbing pain. Tiny red fang marks, slight swelling, difficult to see. Pain increases 1–3 hours, subsides in 12–48 hours.	Seek medical attention. Ice to reduce pain and decrease rate of venom absorption. Muscle relaxants, antivenom, observe carefully. Treatment is symptom related.

(Table 4 Continued on p. 90)

*Black widow and brown recluse spiders are the only spiders in the U.S. which threaten life.

TABLE 4 Continued

WHAT IS SEEN	WHAT TO DO
Rigidity and spasm of large muscle groups.	
Severe abdominal pain not relieved by sedatives and narcotics	
Board-like abdomen	
Progressive muscle pain	
CNS symptoms	
Restless	
May be expiratory grunt	
Elevated temperature and blood pressure	
Elevated WBC	
Oliguria, proteinuria, hematuria	
Elevated CSF pressure	

Brown Recluse

Local

Little pain, early	Seek medical assistance at once.
Severe pain in 2–8 hr	Treatment is symptom related.
Erythema followed by blister at bite site	Steroids are utilized in severe reaction.
Ischemia induration	Bed rest, cold compresses.
Enlarging ulceration over 3-wk period	

General reaction (24–48 hr):
Fever, chills, malaise, weakness, nausea, vomiting, joint pain, rash, petechiae.
Hematological disturbances, hemaglobinemia, leukocytosis, edema, jaundice, seizures, hemoglobinuria, proteinuria, phlebitis.

patients who react to either house dust extract or to mite extract, but not to both. It is possible that the mite, which grows on desquamated human skin, contributes to the breakdown of the vegetable and animal matter to produce the allergen house dust. Causing some confusion is the fact that the reproductive life of the mite is confined to the colder months when house dust provokes many of its symptoms. In addition, at high altitudes where the mite does not grow, dust is not much of a problem.

Animal Danders. This category includes feathers, cat hair, dog hair, horse hair, wool, cattle hair, mohair, and rabbit hair. Although all of these substances are regarded as notorious offenders, the most frequent and worst offender is cat hair. Dog dander is a close second, and horse dander is the third runner up for offender status. Feathers, horse dander, cattle dander, wool, mohair, and rabbit hair are plentiful in the household. Furniture, carpeting, and bedding are frequently made of pressed animal hairs. Carpet pads, robes, caps, gloves, slippers, clothing, toys, coats, doll hair, and rope can all contain animal dander. There appears to be cross sensitivity between cat hair and mouse hair, between cattle hair and horse hair, and between dog hair and cat hair. The person sensitive to one type of animal dander is usually sensitive to others.

There are a few other household allergens that are important in some individuals, but for the purpose of this discussion they will just be listed. These include cottonseed, flaxseed, kapok, pyrethrum, glues, jute, vegetable gums, and orris root.

Pollens and Molds. Children under one year of age have runny noses and/or asthma only from infections or allergies to food. It is not until after this age that inhalant sensitivity to household allergens develops. Pollen and mold sensitivities rarely develop before age 3 or 4. Their onset may even occur in the eighth decade of life. As stated in the discussion of household allergens, a knowledge of which pollens and molds are present in the atmosphere is necessary in order to interpret what the patient is saying to you. One cannot ask pertinent questions without some knowledge of which pollens are important hay fever and asthma producers. Most pollens that precipitate allergic responses are small and easily blown around.

The rose and the sunflower are entomophilous plants and are pollinated by insects. They have flowers and heavy gummy pollens that stick to bellies of insects. The pollen is not blown far by the wind. Contrary to popular belief they are not hay-fever-producing plants. Corn pollen are 200 micra in diameter compared to the 20 micra of ragweed pollen. Wind can carry corn pollen approximately 20 to 40 feet, whereas ragweed pollen may be blown 180 miles away.

Anemophilous plants are wind-pollenated plants. They are light, buoyant, flowerless, and plentiful. Ragweed, grasses, and tree pollens are examples of anemophilous plants. It has been reported that one acre of ragweed can produce 60 pounds of pollen.

Amphibolous plants, an example of which is the willow tree, are pollinated by both insects and wind and are occasionally significant factors in hay fever and asthma. Sensitive persons may be relieved or stressed by a move from one neighborhood to another.

Mold spores are present throughout the warm months of the year, and they can be anywhere in the atmosphere. Spores are also present during a thaw following a killing frost in October and November. In the desert heat or solid winter, molds are almost absent from the atmosphere.

Farmers, furriers, bakers, florists, janitors, barbers, and beauticians all engage in occupations where inhalant-associated allergens have been associated with allergic reactions.

ASTHMATIC REACTIONS

Genetic Factors.   The asthmatic patient may inherit many abnormalities or just a few. These abnormalities are classified as hypoactive beta-adrenergic receptor systems, atopic factors (IgE), aspirin sensitivity or trigger mechanisms (e.g., vagus, alpha-adrenergic, guanosene monophosphate [GMP]).

Types of Asthmatic Reactions.   The classification of astromatic reactions is based on this delineation of abnormalities, with the probability that an underactive beta-adrenergic receptor system and reactions to trigger mechanisms are common to all types of asthmatic reactions. The types of asthma are atopic asthma (IgE), aspirin-sensitive asthma with nasal polyps, intrinsic asthma (unknown cause), and various combinations of each.

Trigger Mechanisms.   Trigger mechanisms are not allergens. They aggravate the tracheobronchial tree so that it becomes more edematous, and bronchospasms are also produced. Many trigger mechanisms are mediated through the vagus nerve and the alpha-adrenergic system. The action of these mediators has been blocked by the administration of large doses of atropine. The following is a list of common trigger mechanisms.

Possible Trigger Mechanisms

Infection
Physical exertion
Changes in barometric pressure, wind, rain, cold air
Paint, hay, moth balls, floor wax, insecticides, sprays, perfumes
Smoke
Emotions
Oil of wintergreen and similar irritants rubbed on the chest for colds
Alcohol

Exertion and cold air increase guanosene monophosphate (GMP), which causes a decrease in cyclic adenosene monophosphate (CAMP). When CAMP levels are decreased, there is an increased release of histamine and slow-reacting substance (SRS) from the mast cells. This is in essence the mechanism that triggers the asthmatic episode.

Bacterial Allergy. The area of bacterial allergy has been an area of controversy for a long time. There are those who believe that there is an interaction resulting in allergy, but in at least seven double-bind studies, this assumption has been proven false. However, it has been proven that infections can reduce CAMP levels resulting in histamine and slow-reacting substance release from the mast cells.

In general, any substance that you can smell or that is the least bit irritating to the mucous membranes has the potential to act as a trigger mechanism in asthma. Thus, paint, woodburning fireplaces, Christmas trees, cosmetics, floor wax, and smoke are all suspect.

MANAGEMENT

The management of inhalant and trigger mechanisms in essence is the avoidance of these mechanisms whenever possible. Hyposensitization therapy is also sometimes useful.

Household Allergens. Although precaution in the entire household is a superhuman task, the bedroom, where the patient sleeps and spends one-third to one-half of his lifetime, lends itself well to the application of the avoidance concept. The mattress, box spring, and pillows should be enclosed in impervious plastic, which is available in most bedding stores. No stuffed animals, heavy drapes, or carpet are permitted. A small synthetic throw rug that can be laundered is permitted. Furnace filters should be changed every two weeks in the winter months. The bed should not be placed in the direct draft of a forced air heating system. If possible, close all registers and have the bedroom heated by the rest of the house. The placement of damp cheese cloth over the register will help catch dust. This should be changed and laundered daily.

House plants are dust and mold producers and should be removed. Mold present in a home can be reduced for up to six months by placing a coffee can containing a thin layer of formaldehyde in each room of the house when the family goes on vacation.

Pollens and Molds. There are a few simple concepts related to outdoor pollens and molds that are significant. A bedroom with an air conditioner provides an excellent haven for the patient. It can reduce outdoor pollen levels from 100 percent outdoors to 10 percent in the bedroom. Windy night air should be avoided, and the wearing of glasses will prevent pollen from hitting the eyeballs. Application of plain vaseline in each side of the nose with the little finger several times a day will trap pollen and mold granules at the nasal entrance and prevent absorption by the nasal mucosa. The patient should stay indoors as much as possible, especially on windy days.

Nursing Role. The nursing role in the care of the allergic patient, in addition to assisting with the provision of medical therapy, is in the area of prophylaxis. Every attempt should be made to eliminate as many food, inhalant, and triggering factors as possible. There are many problems in dealing with asthmatic patients, and there are still unanswered questions and no easy solutions. Many treatment failures are related to inadequate patient and family cooperation. This includes smokers, pets, and inability or inadequacy of the persons involved to avoid inhalant and dietary allergens.

Allergic Tension Fatigue Syndrome

There is one additional topic that seems worthy of mentioning in this chapter, the allergic tension fatigue syndrome. It has a controversial place in the literature, and the authors wish to alert the reader to the issues involved, without attempting to either substantiate or refute related findings.

The allergic tension fatigue syndrome has been described by many physicians. However, it is continually overlooked or ignored by many others who do not believe it exists. Common manifestations of the allergic syndrome are pallor, infraorbital circles, nasal stuffiness, fatigue, irritability, headache, abdominal pain, and muscle aches and pains. More severe and bizarre systemic and nervous system symptoms such as hyperactivity, learning problems, and obsessive compulsive symptoms have also been reported.

Children with this syndrome often have the typical allergic look, which consists of dull facies, pallor, infraorbital circles, and "allergic gape." The physical assessment is normal in other areas. Blood counts, x-rays, and allergy skin tests are normal.

Theorists believe that the syndrome is caused by common foods, but may also be caused by drugs, food coloring, and other additives, inhaled pollens, dusts, chemical fumes, and other odoriferous substances. The questions that evolve around the validity of this syndrome can only be answered when health care providers are sufficiently aware of the possibility of its existence. The alleviation of symptoms subsequent to an elimination diet that reappear when identified offenders are eaten again will at least give clinical support to its existence.

There are investigators who believe that this syndrome, along with other types of systemic allergic reactions, is one of the most common causes of physical and emotional illness seen in ambulatory child health care settings.

Type II: Cytotoxic Reactions

Type II reactions are caused by antibodies that react with antigens on the membranes of cells. Common examples of this phenomenon are hemolytic anemia and thrombocytopenia. These reactions are sometimes provoked by drugs. The affected cells are taken up in the reticuloendothelial system or are lysed by complement.

IMMUNE CYTOLYSIS OF ERYTHROCYTES

There are two types of cytolysis resulting from immune reactions directly against the erythrocyte, warm-type cytolysis and cold-type cytolysis. The warm-type immune cytolysis of erythrocytes is not necessarily complement dependent. It is usually mediated by IgG-type autoantibody. Cold-type antierythrocyte autoantibodies directed against red cells require colder temperatures and are mainly IgM autoantibodies.

Warm-type Immune Cytolysis. In many types of acquired hemolytic anemia, erythrocyte antigens to which autoantibody is directed are antigens of the Rh system other than Rh_o(D). The IgG antibodies not specific to Rh are usually associated with the binding of complement to red blood cells. In drug-induced hemolytic anemia the IgG autoantibodies are usually involved; however, other classes of immunoglobins may be involved. In penicillin-related hemolytic disease the autoantibody is directed at the penicillin, whereas in alpha-methyldopa-related hemolytic anemia the autoantibody is directed against the red cell itself. It is possible for red cells, white cells, and platelets to be lysed as a result of immune complex formation. Drugs associated with this type of reaction are quinidine, quinine, and stibophen. In this reaction there is a formation of a drug antibody complex. This complex is capable of binding complement at the surface of the cell.

The main mechanism for red cell destruction is erythrocyte fragmentation Erythrophagocytosis occurs via the macrophages in the spleen, liver, bone marrow, and at times, the lymph nodes are involved. When hyperplasia of the reticuloendothelial system and lymphatic system occurs, as in mononucleosis, autoimmune hemolytic disease due to warm-type autoantibodies may occur.

Hemolytic disease due to warm-type autoantibody formation may occur at any age. This disorder is not common in children, but the incidence increases with age. There has been a higher reported incidence in postmenopausal women. It is possible for autoimmune hemolytic disease to occur idiopathically and it may

occur in association with malignancies such as chronic lymphocytic leukemia.

Cold-Type Autoantibody Reactions. The cold-type antibodies
agglutinate red cells at between 0 to 5 C and are not capable of
causing hemolysis at temperatures above 30 C. This is the reason
that in the human system there is little opportunity for cold agglu-
tinization to occur. It is possible that during cold weather the
temperature in exposed parts of the body such as the face, hands,
and toes may reach 28 to 31 C. During this period cold agglutinins
are capable of binding to erythrocytes. IgM immune cytolysis is
complement dependent, and the action of the complement cascade occurs only at temperatures above 37 C. Thus for this type of
cytolysis to occur, the affected person must first be exposed to
cold and then returned to a warmer environment. The degree of
reaction in relation to temperature exposure is variable. In some
patients massive reactions occur after minor chilling, and in others
more extreme temperature variation is required to initiate a reaction. Reactions occur within minutes to hours after an exposure,
and the hemolysis is acute and intermittent. The major mechanisms
of red cell destruction is the same as in the warm-type autoantibody hemolytic disorder. There is fragmentation and subsequent
erythrophagocytosis.

Cold-type antibodies of the IgG class have also been reported.
They are called the cold hemolysins and also activate complement.

In patients with mycoplasma pneumonia a transitory elevation
of the cold agglutinins of the IgM class occurs. In patients with
mononucleosis cold-reactive antierythrocyte antibodies of the IgG
class are found. The cold hemolysin syndrome is also seen in idiopathic or late syphilis, and transiently in virus infections. Individuals with chronic cold agglutinin disease may, on electrophoresis,
exhibit a homogenous IgM spike. This should not be confused
with Waldenstroms' macroglobulinemia.

CYTOTOXICITY DIRECTED AT CELLS
OTHER THAN ERYTHROCYTES

Antibody-mediated cytotoxicity injury is caused by immunoglobulins bound to monocyte membranes. This type of reaction also
requires complement activation. The target cell may be any cell

displaying membrane antigens against which the antibody is specifically directed. The ability for T cells to destroy cells and mediate autoimmune injury in humans is still an area of controversy. T cells are cytotoxic in vitro. Antibody-mediated cytotoxic phenomena are beneficial if directed against a tumor cell, but harmful if the target is a normal cell or allograft.

Type III: Immune-Complex-Mediated Injury

This type of hypersensitivity reaction was initially described by Arthus, and its local manifestation is sometimes called an Arthus reaction. It is dependent on the formation of immune complexes of antibody and antigen. These immune complexes fix complement and result in the release of vasoactive substances leading to local vascular lesions, or if they enter the circulation serum sickness (a syndrome composed of fever, joint pain, urticaria, and proteinuria) may result. The systemic reaction results from the effect of inflammatory mediators released after complement activation. Polymorphonuclear leukocytes (PMNs) are attracted to this phenomena and in their attempt to clear up the deposits resulting from this reaction they digest portions of the basement membrane. This permits the passage of blood cells and serum proteins into tissues, urine, and joints.

LOCAL REACTION VERSUS SYSTEMIC REACTIONS

In local Arthus reactions antigen is injected intradermally into persons with high antibody titers. In the systemic reaction (serum sickness), antigen is injected intramuscularly or intravenously and diffused into general circulation. Reactions occur within four to six hours after antigenic stimulation. Hemorrhagic necrosis is common to both reactions. The characteristic local manifestation is an area of hemorrhage surrounded by erythema. The hemorrhagic necrosis resulting from the systemic reaction can lead to shock and death subsequent to necrosis of the circulatory vasculature. The reaction has usually peaked in 24 to 36 hours.

FARMERS' LUNG

Farmers' lung is considered a Type III immune-complex-mediated hypersensitivity reaction. Dust-borne fungal spores are inhaled, and in six to eight hours the antigen reacts with IgG in the lung. An inflammatory reaction results, and larger amounts of IgG appear, as well as complement-fixing IgA. This reaction also explains the allergy called pigeon-fanciers disease, which is caused by an inhalant antigen thought to be a serum protein from dried bird feces.

SERUM SICKNESS

Serum sickness occurs as the result of injections of antigenic protein. It is seen following the administration of animal sera antitoxin. This phenomenon occurs 7 to 10 days after the administration of the antigenic protein substance. The acute form of the reaction is IgE mediated, and the chronic form of the disorder is due to an immune complex reaction. The chronic symptoms of joint pain and kidney stones result from the deposition of the immune complex in these areas.

VIRUS-ANTIBODY COMPLEXES

Complexes of virus-antibody, and even soluble tumor antigen-antibody, have been reported to induce immune complex mediated hypersensitivity in rare cases. The resulting injury commonly affects the glomeruli.

POST-BETA-HEMOLYTIC STREPTOCOCCAL GLOMERULONEPHRITIS

Glomerulonephritis secondary to a beta-hemolytic streptococcal infection is assumed to develop from the passage of soluble antigen-antibody complexes through the pores of the endothelium into the basement membrane, where they form deposits. In an attempt to reach these deposits the PMN digests a portion of the basement membrane. This permits the passage of blood cells and protein into the urine. Antibody-antigen complexes are no longer produced when the supply of antigen is used up, and therefore the disorder is usually self limiting.

GOODPASTURE'S SYNDROME

In Goodpasture's syndrome the action of the antigen-antibody complex is directed against the glomerular basement membrane itself, where IgG and C_3 are deposited. When the immune complex is related to the glomerular membrane rather than the nephritogenic streptococci, as in the poststreptococcal immune complex disorder, the disease is not self limiting. The IgG secreted from the kidney in Goodpasture's syndrome is directed against the basement membrane antigens of the glomeruli, and antibodies from the kidney or lungs will continue to bind the basement membranes either in the kidney or pulmonary alveoli.

SYSTEMIC LUPUS ERYTHEMATOSUS (SLE)

The syndrome associated with systemic lupus erythematosus results from the formation of immune complexes. There is resulting kidney damage, central nervous system involvement, and skin rash.

Type IV: Cell-Mediated Delayed Hypersensitivity

Type IV reactions depend upon the sensitization of mononuclear cells. These cells react with antigen in the sensitized area. There is a release of lymphokines (factors that affect cell permeability and the signaling and activation of macrophages and other factors involved in the inflammatory response). This reaction is exemplified by the tuberculin skin test and characterizes infections of the lung (e.g., pulmonary tuberculosis). Skin disorders such as contact dermatitis, which develop subsequent to repeated exposure to a sensitizing substance, are examples of delayed hypersensitivity reactions. This type of response also occurs in disorders resulting from autoimmune reactions, such as ulcerative colitis and Hashimoto's thyroiditis.

TYPES OF REACTIONS

The significance of cell-mediated immune injury is being actively
studied at this time. There are actually three types of reactions
that take place: initiation of an allograft rejection, graft versus
host reaction, and the delayed hypersensitivity reaction. Sensitized
lymphocytes (T lymphocytes) interact with antigen in this reaction and initiate the release of the lymphokines. Injury results
from the action of the lymphotoxin on the target cell or by direct
interaction between the T cell membrane and the antigen of the
target cell.

Most contact dermatitis is a Type IV reaction. The role of established mechanisms of immunological injury is still unclear in some
disorders termed autoimmune phenomena, such as rheumatic
fever. Some investigators feel that all organ-specific autoimmunity
can be initiated by T cells in the same way that an allograft rejection occurs.

Type V: Antibody-Mediated Stimulation

Antibody-mediated stimulation has been proposed as a mechanism
of immune injury. This would be a Type V reaction. In this reaction, antibody stimulates target cells to overproduce normal
products. There is presently only one example of this type of
phenomenon, Grave's disease or thyrotoxicosis. The antibody
involved is an IgG also called long-acting thyroid stimulator
(LATS). This antibody affects the membrane of the thyroid cells
in a manner similar to thyroid-stimulating hormone (TSH, which
stimulates T_4 and T_3 production). The pituitary-thyroid axis
has no control over the LATS, and overproduction results in
thyrotoxicosis.

AUTOIMMUNE PHENOMENON

In autoimmune reactions the immune system sees the self as
antigenic. Autoimmune reactions, either T or B cell mediated,
result from alterations in self antigens, a deficient immune system,

or a combination of both factors. It is possible for autoantibodies to be present in an individual without the presence of autoimmune disease. The term autoimmune reaction implies that structural or functional damage results from the interaction of T and/or B cells and normal components of the body.

The incidence of autoimmune disease increases with age. It is more common in females than in males, and more frequent in persons with malignancies and immunodeficiency disorders. It is not uncommon for more than one autoimmune disorder to occur in the same individual. There is controversy regarding whether the susceptibility to autoimmune phenomena is inheritable. It has been reported to occur in several members of the same family.

Types

Autoimmune diseases are categorized by some theorists as follows:

Generalized
1. Rheumatoid arthritis
2. Acquired autoimmune hemolytic anemia
3. Systemic lupus erythematosus
4. Idiopathic thrombocytopenia purpura

Organ specific
1. Hashimoto's thyroiditis
2. One type of thyrotoxicosis
3. Allergic encephalitis
4. Allergic neuritis
5. Allergic orchitis and aspermatogenesis
6. Uveitis
7. Myasthenia gravis
8. Pernicious anemia
9. Addison's disease

Altered Self Antigens
1. Heterogenetic Antigens
   a. Poststreptococcal sequelae (rheumatic fever, glomerulo-nephritis)
   b. Gram-negative enteritis
2. Drug induced
   a. Certain purpuras
   b. Penicillin (hemolytic anemia)

Etiological Mechanisms

The etiological mechanism behind autoimmune phenomena is controversial. It has been hypothesized that the T cell loses its suppressor activity for antigen recognition as a result of the aging process. This implies that antibody synthesis is dependent on the interaction of both the T and B systems, and that immune tolerance occurs if the antigen binds to only one type of cell. Theorists believe that induction of antibodies to thymic antigens occurs before the production of other antoantibodies. They propose that T cells develop responses against B cell antigens. Viruses are the agents proposed to alter thymic antigenicity. In patients with immunodeficiency diseases the presence of autoantibodies is theoretically due to the lack of suppression from the T cell population.

Viruses

Virsues are considered to be the agents most likely to induce autoimmune disease. They appear to be capable of altering the immunological apparatus, as well as modifying self antigens. Autoimmune disease may occur following a viral infection during which the virus has altered the immune apparatus. An immune complex is formed by the virus and antibody, which results in a Type III hypersensitivity reaction. The antibody and complement formed may then interact with virus-induced cell surface antigens, and a Type II hypersensitivity reaction results. Lastly, there may be interaction between the T cells and macrophages, with infected and altered cells resulting in a Type IV hypersensitivity reaction.

There are groups of viruses called slow viruses which require prolonged periods of incubation and result in a protracted disease course after they become clinically visible. The outcome of diseases caused by these viruses is serious and often ends in death. Agents such as slow viruses may alter the self cell antigens because of their persistence within the cell.

Some investigators believe that there is an antecedent viral infection associated with the genesis of diabetes mellitus in humans. Investigators have reported the presence of autoantibodies in patients with myasthenia gravis. In addition, evidence now exists which indicates that immune T cells with thyroid antigen are involved in Hashimoto's thyroiditis and Graves' disease.

Bacteria

Autoimmune phenomena have been associated with a variety of microbial diseases (e.g. tuberculosis, syphilis, gonorrhea). Even malaria, a protozoan-borne infection has been related to the development of autoantibodies.

Some investigators believe that autoimmune diseases are really a form of immundeficiency disorder. This is hypothetically related to a deficiency of secretory IgA. However, many people with an intact secretory immunoglobin system develop autoimmune disease. It is well accepted that persons with deficiencies in complement components are not only more susceptible to infection, but also to autoimmune diseases.

Malignancy and Autoimmune Disease

The relationship of malignancy and autoimmune disease probably occurs because susceptibility to a single disease is controlled by many genes. Some HL-A types are associated with an increased risk of developing Hodgkin's disease, chronic glomerulonephritis, systemic lupus erythematosus, acute lymphoblastic leukemia, lymphomas, psoriasis, and ankylosing spondylitis. These cause-effect relationships are not completely accepted by many investigators.

Drugs

There are many drugs, the antibiotics in particular, that are able to induce allergy. They have been associated with all four types of allergic reactions. Certain antiepileptic drugs cause abnormal alterations in lymphoid tissue and are reported to initiate or facilitate reoccurrence of active disease in systemic lupus erythematosus patients. This disease may also be exacerbated by unrelated drugs such as sulfa and penicillin.

MALIGNANCY: IMMUNOLOGICAL ENHANCEMENT

Immunological emhancement is the most widely accepted hypothesis brought forward to explain the progression of tumor growth. This concept refers to the presence of antibody that coats and protects tumor cells from destruction by the host's immunological system.

Tumor Antigens

Most, if not all, tumors possess distinctive antigens on their cell surfaces which are capable of evoking both cell-mediated and low antibody responses. It has been hypothesized that one of the major functions of the immune system is the surveillance of foreign cells and prevention of their progression to neoplastic disease. Much of what is known today regarding this surveillance phenomenon is based on animal research. Tumor cells exhibit a new cell surface antigen, which can be located by the lymphoid cells responsible for contacting and eliminating them. These antigens are classified as virally induced, embryonic, divisional, and idiotypic.

Virally Induced Antigens

Our knowledge of virally induced antigens is based on animal research. Some human viruses have been proven to cause cancer in animals. Oncogenic viruses have on their cell surface a new antigen called tumor specific transplantation antigen (TSTA) or tumor specific antigen (TSA). All tumors produced by a given virus will carry this specific cell surface antigen regardless of the morphology of the organ in which the tumor is present. Some theoretical formulations drawn from this hypothesis propose that immunization specifically directed at TSA would destroy the tumor cells and have no harmful effect on the host, because the antigenic determinant would be found only on cells with the TSA antigen. Some researchers believe that this type of immunization could confer immunity against the challenge of other tumors caused by the same virus. The possibility of using TSA level assays for diagnostic purposes also has been suggested. However, the role of the virus as a human etiological oncogenic agent is still speculative. The only malignant disease in man known to be of viral origin in Burkitt's lymphoma, which is due to Epstein-Barr virus. Many of these clinical possibilities have yet to be related to actual practice, but they do suggest some challenging possibilities for the future.

Embryonic Antigens

Tumors in humans arising from the same cell type have cell-surface differentiative antigens that are also found on embryonic cells. The first of these is carcinoembryonic antigen (CEA), which is associated with cancer of the gastrointestinal tract. CEA is discarded from the tumor cell and can be detected in the serum of patients with gastrointestinal cancers. The host immune response to this antigen is presently under study.

Another fetal antigen is alpha-fetoprotein, which is found in patients with hepatoma and teratocarcinoma of the testes and ovaries. Asia and Africa have the highest incidence of this type of cancer. The infant halts synthesis of this antigen shortly after birth, and serum detection would be indicative of oncogenic transformation.

Divisional Antigens

It is postulated that cell surface antigens may change during early mitosis. These antigens would be termed divisional antigens. It is believed that some oncofetal antigens are a form of divisional antigen. Theorists believe this type of divisional antigen can be considered a possible source of tumor development.

Idiotypic Antigens

This group consists of chemical carcinogens, i.e., hydrocarbons that are thought to possess specific TSA. They differ from virus-induced tumors in that each tumor produced by a chemical has its own individual idiotypic antigen, even if it produces two different primary tumors in the same animal.

Physiological Considerations

The physiological variations at the extremes of life's continuum must be considered. The newborn's immune response is structurally complete but functionally immature. This could have some influence on the incidence of embryonic tumors in infancy. The functionally immature infant is also more susceptible to infection, and the possibility of cellular alteration due to an infection-producing organism is increased.

Immunological function undergoes deterioration in senescence resulting in an increased rate of malignancy, autoimmune disease, antibody deficiency, impaired delayed hypersensitivity reactions, and the slowing of lymphocyte proliferation.

Finally, there appears to be an increased incidence of neoplastic diseases in patients with immunodeficiency diseases. Some examples are ataxia-telangiectasis, Wiskott-Aldrich syndrome, Down's syndrome, Bloom's syndrome, and the Chediak-Higashi syndrome.

Transplants

Neoplasms have been transferred to the transplant recipient in about 1 percent of renal transplant patients. Generally this tumor is of the reticuloendothelial system. Cessation of immunosuppressive therapy has resulted in the rejection of the tumor as well as the graft. However, it may not lead to tumor rejection in the presence of an enhancing antibody.

Conclusion

Many efforts are being made to manipulate the immune response, although most have been unsuccessful to date. The oncologist wishes to find a way to help the host mount an adequate immune response that "kills" the tumor, to find an immunization to boost the response if the T cell system is ineffective, and to find a way to suppress enhancing antibody if these antibodies are interfering with immunological success.

SUGGESTED READINGS

Baer RL, Harber LC: Reactions to light, heat, and trauma. In Samter M (ed): Immunological Diseases, 2nd ed. Boston, Little Brown, 1971
Becker EL: Nature and classification of immediate-type allergic reactions. Adv Immunol 13:267, 1971

Cochrane CG, Dixon FJ: Cell and tissue damage through antigen-antibody complexes. In Miescher PA et al (eds): Textbook of Immunopathology. New York, Grune and Stratton, 1968

Cochrane CG, Koffler D: Immune complex diseases in experimental animals and man. Adv Immunol 16:186, 1973

Crook G: The allergic tension fatigue syndrome. Pediatr Ann 3:69–77, 1976

Crook WC: Recurrent Abdominal Pain. Pediatrics 46:969, 1970

Deamer WC: Recurrent abdominal pain: a frequent manifestation of food allergy. CMD 40:130–154, 1973

——: Environmental control in treatment of atopic diseases. In Kelley VC (ed): Practice of Pediatrics. Hagerstown, Md., Harper, 1973, Vol. 2, Chap 73

——: Techniques of desensitization therapy. Primary care 1:87, 1974

——: Injection therapy. Pediatr Ann 3:56–77, 1976

Frazier CA: Insect Allergy: Allergic and Toxic Reactions to Insects and Other Arthropods. St. Louis, Warren H Green Inc., 1975

——: A guide to insect bites and stings. Pediatr Basics 15: 14–15, 1976.

Frick OL: Immunopharmacologic mechanisms in allergy. Pediatr Ann 3:92–108, 1976

Galant SP: The inhibitory effect of anti-allergic drugs on allergen and histamine-induced wheal and flare response. J Allergy Clin Immunol 51:11, 1973

Galant SP et al: An immunological approach to the diagnosis of food sensitivity. Clin Allergy 3:353, 1973

Gerrard JW: Allergy in infancy. Pediatr Ann 3:9–23, October, 1974

Johansson SGO: IgE and allergic asthma. In Reed CE, Siegel SC (eds): Asthma. New York, Medcom, 1974

Johansson SGO et al: The clinical significance of IgE. Prog Clin Immunol 1:157, 1972

Johnstone DE, Dutton A: The valve of hyposensitization therapy for bronchial asthma in children—a 14 year study. Pediatrics 42:793, 1968

Kaliner MA et al: Immunological release of histamine and slow reacting substance of anaphylaxis from human lung. J Exp Med 136:556, 1973

Kallin E: Report of the Chairman to Insect Allergy Committee of the American Academy of Allergy. Feb. 4, 1964

Lessof MH: The immunological basis of allergy. The Practitioner 208:735–741, 1976

Minor TE et al: Viruses as precipitants of asthmatic attacks in children. JAMA 227:292–298, 1974

Mueller HL: Stinging insect allergy. Pediatr Ann 3:43–53, 1976

Orange RP, Austen KF: The immunological release of chemical mediators of immediate type hypersensitivity from human lung. In Amos B (ed): Progress in Immunology I. New York, Academic, 1971

Oster J: Recurrent abdominal pain, headache, and limb pain in children and adolescents. Pediatrics 50:429, 1972

Pepys J: Disodium cromoglycate in clinical and experimental asthma. In Austin KF, Lichtenstein LM (eds): Asthma. New York, Academic, 1973

Pepys J: Hypersensitivity diseases of the lungs due to fungi and ogranic dusts. In Kallos P et al (eds): Monographs in Allergy, vol 4. Basel, Karger, 1969

Peters DK: The immunological basis of glomerulonephritis. Proc Ray Soc Med 67:557, 1974

Randolph TG: Allergy as a causative factor of fatigue, irritability and behavior problems of children. J Pediatr 31:560, 1947

Reed E, Siegel SC (eds): Asthma. New York, Medcom, 1974

Roitt IM: Essential Immunology. Oxford, Blackwell, 1971

Rothfield N et al: Glomerular and dermal deposition of properdin in systemic lupus erythematosus. N Engl J Med 287:681, 1972

Savilohti E: Immunoglobulin-containing cells in the intestinal mucosa and immunoglobulin in the intestinal juice of children. Clin Exp Immunol 11:415, 1972

Shaffer JH: Stinging insects—a threat to human life. JAMA 177:477, 1961

Speer F: The allergic tension fatigue syndrome. Pediatr Clin N Am 1:1029, 1954

Sunshine P et al: Intractable diarrhea in infancy. Relationship to a severe gastrointestinal allergy. Clin Res 20:257, 1972

Turk JL: Immunology in clinical medicine. New York, Appleton, 1969

CHAPTER EIGHT

Nursing Implications of Immunological Concepts

There are still large numbers of children dying from diseases that they never should have developed. Others are affected by complications of such diseases, including blindness, deafness, and brain damage. There are even a number of adults who succumb to conditions for which prevention is already available.

These realities provide a challenge for nurses and other members of the health team to recommit themselves to immunization programs and to creatively facilitate their administration. Safe vaccines are now available for a large number of diseases, but there seems to be an attitude prevalent in society that these diseases are only historical fantasies. It has been reported that vaccination levels in the United States are dangerously low. In the past year, the collaborative efforts of various health disciplines have furthered community awareness and reassessed and developed programs directed toward prevention of adequate health care in this area.

The first section of this chapter deals with the immunological concepts that form the scientific basis for practice in this area. Nursing personnel are frequently involved in leadership roles in the planning and administration of such programs, and this information provides the rationale on which decisions regarding physiological implications of such programs should be made. This is fundamental to the nursing process and the moral responsibilities inherent in a professional role.

The second section of the chapter deals with another type of therapy resulting from the application of immunological concepts, i.e., immunotherapy. This concept has gained wider application in recent years and will probably be one of the major therapies of the future. An assessment of available approaches and therapeutic application is provided as well as an indication of areas where controversy exists at present.

The last section of this chapter describes environmental variables that have been identified as significant to the maintenance of immunological function. Knowledge of these variables should alert the nurse to patients at risk in immunological terms. These patients have a higher probability of exhibiting decreased ability to cope with immunological stressors, stressors that normal persons could easily adapt to without a disease state resulting. This whole area of environmental variables has wide application in nursing practice, as the nursing process requires the identification of potential stressors and is directed toward the prevention of disease and maintenance of the health state.

IMMUNIZATIONS

Immunizations are a means of providing protection, either temporary or permanent, against stress from immunogenic agents. The term vaccination is frequently used synonymously with immunization. An antigen used to immunize is called a vaccine. There are two types of immunity provided by immunization, active and passive. Immunization either provides protection against disease or limits the severity of the disease process.

There are several factors that determine the effectiveness of a vaccine: its antigenic components, the route of administration, the dose given, the time at which the vaccine is given, the immunological competence of the vaccinated individual, and the potential side effects associated with the immunizing antigen. All of these factors are considered when preparing recommendations regarding optimal immunization programs.

Immunizations may begin at any age but usually are initiated at the age of two months. This process continues throughout child-hood, with booster doses dependent on the specific vaccine utilized. Factors that are considered when planning for booster doses are the type of vaccine utilized, the desired length of protection, and the length of protection provided by immunization with a particular variety of vaccine. Interruptions in the immunization process never necessitate extra doses or initiating the immunization process again. Once specificity is determined (ability to react to a specific antigen), the length of time between challenges does not alter the quality of the final immunity.

General Principles

All depot antigens, such as diphtheria-pertussis-tetanus (DPT) should be injected directly into muscle, and each dose should be given at a different site. Sterile technique is essential, and aspirin or acetaminophen in therapeutic doses (dependent on the subject's weight and age) should be utilized to minimize discomfort subsequent to the administration of the antigen.

Contraindications

Several general principles clearly prohibit the administration of a vaccine. Immunizations should be withheld if an acute febrile illness is present (temperature elevation greater than 101 F [38.3 C]). A minor upper respiratory infection is not sufficient reason in itself to contraindicate the administration of a vaccine. Immuno-suppression therapy is another prohibiting factor. The administration of gamma globulin, plasma, or a blood transfusion with the preceding six to eight weeks negates the effectiveness of vaccination. If a live vaccine is administered, additional live vaccines should not be used simultaneously unless this procedure has been tested and approved. The approved vaccines are usually available in combined form for multivalent administration. The trivalent oral polio vaccine (OPV) and measles, mumps, and rubella (MMR) are examples of such preparations. Live virus vaccines should not be given to pregnant women. Persons with immunological disorders and malignancies are not candidates for immunization. The

DPT vaccine should not be used in persons over six years of age, and those who develop reactions should receive fractional doses of this vaccine when it is next administered, usually one-third of the usual dose on a delayed schedule in an attempt to achieve adequate immunity without initiating a systemic reaction.

Current Data Sources

The Committee on Infectious Disease of the American Academy of Pediatrics publishes a biyearly Red Book that provides approved immunization schedules and information related to use, side effects, and effectiveness of available immunogens. The World Health Organization regularly updates its data regarding required and suggested immunization requirements for those traveling to the United States from other countries and for those Americans wishing to travel to another country.

A current immunization schedule is provided in Table 5. At the present time DPT and OPV vaccinations are initiated at age two months, and two additional doses are provided at two-month intervals. Booster doses of OPV and DPT are given at age 18 months and before entry to school. At age 16 an OPV booster and a dose of adult diphtheria and tetanus vaccine is suggested. Measles, mumps, and rubella vaccines in combined form (MMR) or separately are given at five to eight week intervals after the child's first birthday.

TABLE 5 Recommended Schedule for Active Immunization of Normal Infants and Children*

2 mo	DTP	TOPV
4 mo	DTP	TOPV
6 mo	DTP	TOPV
15 mo	Measles	Tuberculin test
	Rubella	Mumps
1½ yr	DTP	TOPV
4–6 yr	DTP	TOPV
14–16 yr, then every 10 yr	Td	

*DPT: Diptheria, tetanus, pertussis; TOPV: trivalent oral polio; Td: tetanus, diptheria.

The following discussion will consider passive immunizations and common and available active immunization agents. Lastly, a discussion of vaccines currently under development will be included.

Passive Immunization

Passive immunization provides temporary protection from a potential or imminent stressor. Antibodies from subjects competent in dealing with the stressor are given to those who are at risk. Passive immunization is utilized when active vaccines are unavailable or when exposure has occurred and active vaccination is not feasible because too much time has elapsed. The theoretical basis of passive immunization involves developing adequate serum antibody levels in subjects and achieving this level early in the incubation period.

There are two types of preparations from humans used to provide passive immunity: standard human immunoglobulins and special human immune serum globulins. These are identical preparations except that the antibody content is higher in the latter. In addition to the human preparations, animal antisera and antitoxin, usually from the horse, are also utilized. Many persons with an allergic history react to the animal preparations because of prior sensitization. A careful allergy history should be elicited prior to the administration of animal sera. In addition, history regarding prior therapy with animal sera is of utmost importance. If the history is indicative of a probable reaction, the dose of sera may be reduced and/or hypersensitivity screening initiated prior to therapy. Reaction to animal sera are of two types: anaphylactic reactions, which are characterized by urticaria, dyspnea, cyanosis, shock, and unconsciousness within seconds or minutes after injection, and serum sickness reactions, which present hours to days after injections, depending on dose and the presence and/or degree of sensitization. The greater the degree of sensitization the earlier and more severe the reaction. Serum sickness presents as urticaria, arthritis, adenopathy, and fever. Prior to the administration of animal sera, if sensitivity is suspected, scratch and intradermal tests for hypersensitivity should be done. If the results of such tests are negative the sera may be administered intravenously

(IV) or intramuscularly (IM). Special precaution must be used when the animal serum is administered IV. The only reason this type of preparation is used is cost or the lack of available human serum.

The key words are patience, careful observation, and SLOWLY. If skin tests are positive, fractional doses may be attempted or desensitization therapy utilized. Epinephrine should be available at all times. The therapy for anaphylactic shock is related to life-saving measures followed by immunosuppression and avoidance of contact with the antigen in the future.

Active Immunization

Active immunizations routinely used are diphtheria, pertussis, tetanus, poliomyelitis, measles (rubeola), rubella, and mumps.

DIPHTHERIA

The administration of diphtheria toxoid stimulates the production of antitoxin which protects the human organism against harmful effects of disease caused by *Corynebacterium diphtheriae*. The protection is limited to the toxic effects of the disease, not infection itself or carrier states. Immunization schedules presently utilized should provide life-long immunity. The primary series consists of three bimonthly doses and a booster dose one year later. A subsequent booster prior to school entry and at 10-year intervals thereafter is suggested.

The antibody levels developed in the younger infant are not as great as those developed in older infants due to the residual levels of maternal antibody. This does not, however, affect the quality of immunity developed.

Diphtheria toxoid has few associated side effects in the pediatric age range. It is a depot antigen and should be given intramuscularly. The older child and adolescent should receive a reduced dose. This will diminish the possibility of a reaction and still provide adequate immunity.

Passive immunological protection against diphtheria is available. Diphtheria antitoxin is a horse serum preparation. The preparation can be given IV or IM and should be utilized as soon as the clinical diagnosis is made. The dose is related to the level of involvement present, and it appears that the actual dose is less critical than early administration. Sensitivity testing is always required prior to administration, and antibiotic therapy is not a substitute for antitoxin therapy.

PERTUSSIS

The administration of pertussis vaccine provides protection in 80 to 85 percent of the cases. The T cell system is thought to be involved in the development of immunity. This hypothesis is based on the finding that partial protection is provided even at low serum antibody levels.

The need for immunization against pertussis is based on the contagious nature of the disease; 90 percent of exposed subjects develop clinical disease. In addition the course is usually severe, especially in young subjects. Adverse reactions subsequent to pertussis immunization have been reported. These reactions are both local and systemic. Central nervous system reactions such as pertussis meningoencephalitis may occur. This reaction can be severe, but is rare. Local and mild systemic reactions are common. These consist of erythema at the site, fever, and irritability. There is an increased possibility of local reaction with each dose. Due to the frequency of local and systemic reactions, most physicians recommend the administration of aspirin following vaccination. The recommended dosage of aspirin is about 75 mg times the year of age, every four hours.

Pertussis vaccine is usually given in combination with diphtheria and tetanus. There are clinicians who believe the pertussis vaccination should be avoided in children with cerebral damage or convulsive disorders because of the possible increased risk of central nervous system complications.

Immunization against pertussis is usually begun at two months. Three bimonthly doses are recommended with a booster dose in one year followed by another dose before entry to school. The initial vaccination series should not be used after six years of age unless risk is involved. In endemic areas vaccination is begun on the second day of life. This is followed by monthly doses at one and two months, booster doses at 8, 9, and 18 months of age, and prior to entry to school. Additional booster doses are given at 8 and 12 years to provide adequate immunity in such areas.

Most pertussis vaccines are depot antigens and are administered IM. If moderate reactions occur which are not associated with central nervous system involvement, the dose should be reduced and given separately from other antigens. The appearance of central nervous system symptoms definitely negates further immunization with pertussis vaccine.

Passive immunity against pertussis is provided through the administration of human pertussis immunoglobulin. There is some question regarding the efficacy of this preparation, since it is probable that antibody administered never reaches the bronchial tree where the site of infection exists.

TETANUS

The administration of tetanus toxoid provides immunity against tetanus in almost 100 percent of immunized persons. This near-perfect result in immunity, coupled with the facts that there is no natural immunity to tetanus and antibiotic therapy is ineffective once the clinical disease presents, provides the rationale behind the recommendation that tetanus immunization be given to all individuals.

Tetanus toxin does not cause many side effects in infants and children. A phenomenon similar to an Arthus reaction has been reported in individuals who have received repeated doses of tetanus toxoid. This reaction is related to high antibody titers.

Booster doses after the initial series are recommended every 10 years. This recommendation is based on the fact that titers of antitoxin subsequent to the primary tetanus immunization last for at least 20 years. A memory response accounts for a production of antibody in response to antigen challenge even without booster toxoid.

Tetanus is usually given in combination with diphtheria and pertussis. Three doses are given at bimonthly intervals beginning at two months of age, with a booster dose in one year and before entering school. Boosters at 10-year intervals thereafter provide adequate immunity. Reactions to tetanus vaccine are rare in children, and those that occur are primarily local erythema and tenderness. The possibility of intensified reaction increases with subsequent doses, but this risk can be decreased by reducing the amount of toxoid given.

Human, equine, and bovine tetanus antitoxins are available. However, the use of passive immunization in exposed nonimmune individuals appears valuable only prior to the appearance of clinical disease. The human tetanus immunoglobulin is the preparation of choice. It has almost no side effects and provides prolonged antitoxin levels.

POLIOMYELITIS

Live attenuated vaccines provide the best protection against infection from polio virus. This is due to the fact that this preparation follows the natural route of the disease and stimulates antibody production both at secretory and serum levels. This is necessary in that these two levels of immunity are both essential to provide optimal protection against this virus. The secretory level provides protection against invasion through the gastrointestinal tract, and the serum level provides protection at the systemic level. The absence of protection at the secretory level could result in potential spread of infection to nonimmunized individuals. Immunization with the trivalent oral vaccine provides longlasting (10-year to life) bilevel protection against all three strains of virus.

A poliomyelitis-like illness was reported subsequent to the mass use of OPV Type 3 and Type 1. Controversy exists as to whether this was actually a vaccine-related poliomyelitis. However, these cases, coupled with data regarding increased neuro virulence of Type 3 vaccine, has led to the recommendation that adults should not receive the primary OPV immunization series if they reside in areas where poliomyelitis is not endemic or epidemic.

It should be kept in mind when immunizing young children who are breast fed that poliomyelitis neutralization antibody is contained in the colostrum and breast milk of nursing mothers. There is a possibility that the ingestion of this antibody will interfere with the successful development of immunity, especially in young infants. The suspension of breast feeding for six hours prior to and after OPV vaccination appears to alleviate this phenomenon.

The primary immunization series consists of three bimonthly

two-drop doses at two-month intervals (usually given at the same time the DPT vaccination is provided). A booster dose is given after one year and prior to entry to school. The following method may be utilized for older children, those with uncertain previous vaccination, and those who were immunized with inactivated vaccine; two 2-drop doses are given eight weeks apart, followed by booster doses at one year and prior to entry to school if there has been a period of at least one year since the third dose.

The polio vaccine should not be given to persons with immuno-incompetencies, those on immunosuppression therapy, and pregnant women. OPV is not usually given to adults; however, if protection is required due to exposure, travel or occupation, such persons should be immunized.

Passive immunity via the administration of human serum globulin was once given to all exposed individuals when the disease was prevalent. It was felt that the administration of this preparation reduced the possibility of paralytic disease. However, since the development of the trivalent live attenuated vaccine and mass immunization programs, this type of protection has become passé.

RUBEOLA (MEASLES)

The administration of live attenuated measles vaccine will provide immunity in 90 percent of immunized individuals. The T cell system is involved in the provision of successful immunity against measles. Those with incompetent T systems have developed fatal complications to this disease. The immunity subsequent to vaccination is long lasting; the actual duration requires further observation. Earlier, less attenuated preparations had a high incidence of fever and rash. The more attenuated vaccines still produce a febrile reaction 7 to 10 days following the administration of the vaccine, which may require antipyretic therapy. If the less attenuated strains are utilized the administration of measles immune globulin is of value in reducing the degree of the reaction.

Only one dose of vaccine is required, and this is administered after 15 months of age, usually in combination with rubella and mumps vaccine. If epidemics occur, early vaccination may be required at the age of six months, with a booster dose six months later. Even children with a history of the natural disease should be immunized to ensure adequate antibody response. The vaccination of children at this early age has provoked no additional side effects. As with other vaccines the severity of reactions increases with age. Measles vaccine may be given on the day of exposure to susceptible individuals, and will provide protection in that the incubation period for the natural disease is longer than the time it takes to develop antibodies following the administration of the vaccine. Two or more days following exposure immunization (human measles immune globulin) is indicated, followed by attenuated live virus vaccine in eight weeks.

Measles vaccine should not be given to those with malignancy, immunoincompetency or immunosuppression, active tuberculosis, pregnant women, and those with a history of convulsive disorders. As with all other live virus vaccines, it should not be given eight weeks after the administration of blood, plasma, or immune serum globulin preparations. Antibodies received via these preparations may interfere with the action of this vaccine.

SMALLPOX

There are vaccines available that are not used routinely in the United States at this time. A controversial example is the smallpox vaccine. In the past this preparation was routinely given to all children as a part of the primary immunization series. Recent recommendations are based on the analysis of the relationship between exposure risk and complication risk. At the present time, there is a greater risk of complication from the vaccination than there is from actual exposure to the virus. In addition, due to the relatively long incubation period for the disease, it would be possible to effectively immunize exposed individuals should exposure occur. The incubation period for the natural disease is 30 days, while antibodies following immunization develop within about one week. Thus, protection can be provided by immunization even one week following exposure.

The available vaccine is a live attenuated virus preparation. An attenuated live vaccine is currently being developed and may be of value in the future. The complications following smallpox vaccination include autovaccination to other body parts, vaccinia, eczema, and gangrenous reactions. It is also possible for bacterial superinfection to occur.

Human immune globulin for vaccinia has been proven to be of value in providing passive immunity and in the treatment of some of these side effects. This is most frequently utilized in children who have eczema and require vaccination to travel to an endemic area.

INFLUENZA

There are vaccines available for protection against several strains of influenza virus. In fact, these vaccines are developed almost routinely now to provide protection against changing antigenic forms of virus.

Usually the immunization series consists of two doses two months apart. A booster dose on an annual basis maintains adequate antibody levels. A method of intranasal vaccination has been developed which stimulates the production of secretory IgA. It is felt that immunity results from the production of this secretory antibody because the disease is transmitted via the route of the bronchial tree. The hypothesis is that the antibody in this area will interact with the invading antigen and prevent infection. Only the results of further research in this area will determine the effectiveness of this approach. At present, topical intranasal vaccination is not in general use.

RUBELLA (GERMAN MEASLES)

Immunization with rubella vaccine provides demonstrable serum antibody in about 90 percent of immunized individuals. The T cell system seems to be somehow involved in the provision of immunity against rubella. Rubella vaccination is recommended for all prepubertal children in the United States. This, one hopes, will prevent the disease in these children and will prevent children from carrying the disease to their susceptible mothers. Immunization of adult females, although recommended in England, has several hazards, such as the increased incidence of arthritis and the potential teratogenic effect on an undiagnosed pregnancy.

Although adequate serum antibody levels have been reported in immunized individuals, and protection against the disease has been exhibited, asymptomatic reinfection has occurred in previously immunized individuals. The question regarding the possibility of a reinfected asymptomatic immunized mother transmitting the disease to her fetus remains unanswered. Most researchers believe that this probability is limited since there is no evidence of viremia. While transmission to susceptible individuals has only occurred in a few cases, 75 percent of immunized individuals have recoverable virus in their throats. Researchers feel that the transmission of virus from an immunized child to a pregnant women is unlikely.

There have been a number of side effects reported after the administration of rubella vaccine. As with the other vaccines discussed, the possibility of reaction increases with age. Some of these side effects may occur for as long as 10 days after the administration of the vaccine; 10 to 30 percent of adolescents and adults who receive the vaccine develop a degree of reaction. Side effects are similar to the side effects associated with the natural disease and include arthritis, arthralgia, and peripheral neuritis.

The following questions must arise after the discussion of these problems. Is the virus noted in the throat of immunized individuals contagious? Is mass immunization really effective? And are there significant side effects to be considered? Only further research will provide the answers to these questions. What are the alternatives available? Some theorists suggest the immunization of all pubescent women and the assessment of all women of child-bearing age for the presence of rubella antibody. It is felt that only 15 percent of those of childbearing age would exhibit inadequate titers, and these persons could be immunized if pregnancy were avoided for at least two months. There is still a great deal of controversy among the experts in this area at this time. One should follow protocols established by the Committee on Infectious Disease of The American Academy of Pediatrics, which presently recommends the immunization of all children after one year of age. If the possibility of pregnancy exists, tests should be done prior to immunization to determine if the woman is pregnant; an assessment regarding the presence of adequate antibody levels should be done; and if susceptibility exists without pregnancy an acceptable method of contraception should be used for at least two months following immunization.

PASSIVE IMMUNIZATION AND PREGNANCY

Human serum immune globulin, if administered to susceptible individuals after exposure to rubella, may prevent the development of the rubella rash but not of the infection itself. Studies regarding the use of this preparation in exposed pregnant females indicate that the infants born have had congenital rubella. It is possible that the administration of this preparation may decrease the degree of fetal damage. If exposure occurs early during pregnancy, therapeutic abortion should be considered. The use of human serum globulin is limited to cases where therapeutic abortion is unacceptable.

MUMPS

Immunization with mumps attenuated live virus vaccine provides immunity in 98 percent of immunized individusls without reported side effects. There appears to be life-long immunity following vaccination. There is a measurable response of the T system following immunization. (Mumps is the only common childhood viral infection for which T system immunity can be measured.)

The use of mumps vaccine has gained wider acceptance in recent years. It is frequently given in combination with measles and rubella vaccine to children after 15 months of age. The administration of these vaccines together does not appear to alter the resulting immunity. The administration of the vaccine after exposure to the disease is not useful due to the fact that it takes 28 days to develop antibody, and this is a longer period than the incubation period for the natural disease. The lack of widespread use of the vaccine may be related to the benign nature of mumps in humans.

The administration of this vaccine is not recommended for those with immunodeficiency, those on immunosuppression therapy, or pregnant females. In contrast to the other vaccines discussed, this vaccine is well tolerated by the adult. The use of human immune globulin to provide passive immunity is questionable. It is possible that this preparation may reduce the severity of orchitis in adult males.

TYPHOID

Immunization against typhoid is available, although not routinely used in the United States. It is believed that the vaccine is effective in 50 to 90 percent of cases and is recommended only when one is exposed to a carrier, present during community outbreak, or for foreign travel. It should not be given in the presence of a febrile illness.

RABIES

The vaccine available for protection against rabies is used to immunize exposed individuals. Immunization is possible following exposure due to the relatively long incubation period for the natural disease. The decision to immunize is based on criteria established by the American Academy of Pediatrics and related to the following variables:

1. The species of biting animal
2. The kind of wound
3. The vaccinations status of the biting animal
4. Circumstances of the biting incident
5. Presence of rabies in the area
6. Availability of the biting animal

The vaccine preferred for use is the duck embryo vaccine, although other preparations are available. The vaccination protocol consists of 14 single daily doses. If antirabies serum is given with the rabies vaccine, 20 daily doses plus 2 booster doses within 10 to 20 days following the initial series constitute the primary course.

Reactions to the vaccine are common. These include tenderness, erythema, pruritis, and induration on a local level, and fever and malaise at the systemic level. If neurological reactions occur the immunization procedure must be discontinued.

CHOLERA

Presently available preparations to provide immunity against cholera are of dubious value. Research is being done to develop an oral immunization composed of inactivated bacteria. It is hoped that the immunization following the normal route of entry of the organism will produce secretory IgA levels and a better level of protection.

TUBERCULOSIS

The subject of vaccine to protect humans against tuberculosis (TB) is an interesting one. This vaccine is not routinely given in the United States probably due to the problems that developed early in the history of the vaccine, which were related to poor-quality vaccines with associated fatalities. The development of heat-resistant freeze-dried preparations has overcome much of the variability once associated with TB vaccine preparations. Both attenuated and live vaccines are available for use. Since 1950, the World Health Organization has used BCG (Bacillus Calmette-Guerin) throughout the world to control the spread of TB. Over 250 million persons have been immunized with this preparation without significant side effects. The degree of protection provided has been excellent. Some researchers credit inoculation with BCG with control of certain forms of cancer, control of leprosy, and protection against dermal infections caused by myobacterium ulcerans, as well as tuberculosis. BCG can be given at birth but those older than two months should receive a tuberculin test prior to the administration of the vaccine. This same tuberculin test two or three months following the administration of the vaccine gives evidence of successful immunization if it yields a positive reaction. Further research in this area will probably have an effect on the use of this vaccination in the United States, where presently it is recommended only for certain high-risk groups.

BCG should not be given to immunoincompetent individuals, those in immunosuppression therapy, those with skin infections, and those with burns.

CONCLUSION

Research is constantly being done to develop new and more effective vaccines. A vaccine for pneumococcus infections became available this year. There are vaccines being developed against respiratory viruses, herpes, hepatitis, beta-hemolytic streptococcus, meningococcus, *Pseudomonas aeruginosa,* and shigella. In addition, there are several vaccines available for use that have not been discussed in this chapter. Those who are interested in more information in this area should consult the American Academy of Pediatrics Report of the Committee on Infectious Disease (sometimes known as the Red Book; this publication is updated regularly).

SUPPRESSION OF THE IMMUNE RESPONSE

Suppression of Antibody Production with RhoGAM

It has become possible to suppress antibody production. This process is best exemplified by the RhoGAM program. In this program $Rh_o(D)$ negative mothers are prevented from developing antibodies against $Rh_o(D)$ positive fetal erythrocytes. The RhoGAM contains a high affinity anti-$Rh_o(D)$. This interacts with fetal red cells bearing $Rh_o(D)$ antigen. The $Rh_o(D)$ antigen is present in maternal serum after delivery, in the form of fetal cells that have entered the maternal circulation. The anti-$Rh_o(D)$ acts as an antibody and binds the fetal $Rh_o(D)$ cells preventing stimulation of the maternal immunological response. The bound cells are eventually destroyed by phagocytes. The result of this program is suppression of the production of maternal $Rh_o(D)$ antigen and protection for further offspring against erythroblastosis fetalis. The RhoGAM is human gamma globulin containing $Rh_o(D)$ antibody. It must be given to $Rh_o(D)$ negative mothers with 72 hours of the birth of an $Rh_o(D)$ positive child to prevent antibody production.

Suppression of Antibody Production with 6 Mercaptopurine (6MP)

The preparation 6MP has been used to successfully suppress an immune response. This preparation has inhibited antibody production in transplant and graft patients and prevented rejection reactions.

Desensitization and Hyposensitization

THE PROCESS

Desensitization is a process by which an existing immunological response is limited or totally curtailed. This is by no means a simple task, especially when the memory response of the T and B system is considered.

IgE-mediated hypersensitivity has been treated for many years with a form of desensitization. The hypothesis behind this form of desensitization in humans is that the administration of small amounts of antigen injected over long period of time would stimulate IgG production, and that the patient would utilize this IgG to preferentially bind the antigen and therefore block the lower affinity of IgE from bonding with the antigen. This would inhibit the effect of IgE and prevent an allergic reaction. However, this hypothesis has never been proven and is frequently questioned. Does IgG antibody suppress IgE antibody production? At present clinical evidence is variable and answers, perhaps based on now unknown hypotheses, are in the future.

Temporary. Temporary desensitization has been elicited in animals with severe delayed hypersensitivity reactions and accomplished by the administration of large amounts of antigen. This procedure is effective but only for a short period of time. There are certain diseases that have exhibited a desensitizing effect. Some individuals with Hodgkin's disease and sarcoidosis who had positive skin test reactions have illustrated the loss of this reactivity. Some individuals with fulminating tuberculosis lose the ability to react to tuberculin skin tests. At present the underlying mechanism is not understood, but the phenomenon provides many interesting researchable questions.

Antigenic Matching. Careful attention to the possibility of sensitization should be considered when whole blood transfusions are used. Similarities between donor and recipient should be studied carefully. Prevention of sensitization is attempted by antigenic matching and sometimes by removing cells other than erythrocytes and serum components from the blood. These additional serum components increase the possibility of a reaction and are not therapeutically necessary.

Gamma Globulin. Human globulin has been used to provide antibody for persons with agammaglobulinemia. These individuals with an incompetent B system are unable to resist organisms that do not significantly stress normal persons. The provision of gamma globulin to these persons provides a degree of protection against specific antigens.

TRANSPLANTATION OF IMMUNOCOMPETENCY

Histocompatible Transplants

There are several medical centers that have been able to restore immunocompetency to totally deficient children. This is a relatively new and unique form of therapy that requires well-prepared medical teams, as well as specialized laboratory facilities. The restoration is accomplished through the transplantation of histocompatible (antigenically compatible) stem cells from fetal thymus, liver, bone marrow, or peripheral lymphocytes. The number of children exhibiting T cell, B cell, or combined immunodeficiency has been very small, and major problems in utilizing this type of therapy have been encountered, such as graft versus host reactions. Some of these reactions have been fatal. Considerable research related to these procedures is in progress. Those involved in such research will have much to share in the future. The principles related to care for these patients have just begun to emerge.

Bone Marrow Transplants

The development of multidisciplined bone marrow transplant teams, such as the group at Childrens' Orthopedic Hospital and Medical Center, Seattle, Washington, has resulted in the successful transplantation of bone marrow. There are several steps in this process worthy of consideration. The selection of the donor, compatibility typing, immunosuppression of the recipient, the procedure itself, care of the donor and care of the recipient. Each of these areas will be discussed in the following section.

THE DONOR

A suitable donor must be selected, usually the recipient's sibling. Compatibility is determined based on two laboratory tests, HL-A typing and the mixed leukocyte culture (MLC).

Compatibility Typing. HL-A typing is similar to ABO blood group typing. Each individual has an HL-A type as well as a specific blood group type. The HL-A type is determined by the presence of four antigens. Each individual has a set of four antigens, two from each of their parents. Thus, parents are not suitable donors as they have at least two different antigens than each of their children. The process by which individual antigens are inherited for a family is described in Figure 9. More than 30 HL-A antigen types have already been identified, making the possibility of locating two genetically unrelated individuals with matching antigens only a remote possibility.

The possibility of a perfect match is increased by a second typing analysis. This analysis is the mixed lymphocyte culture (MLC). Lymphocytes of donor and recipient are combined and any significant activity in the culture represents a mismatch. Mismatches are called positive cultures; a match is designated by a negative culture.

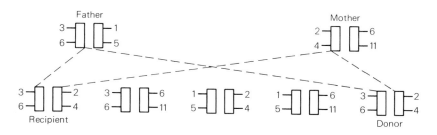

FIGURE 9 HL-A antigens in a family. The rectangles represent chromosomes, the numbers the antigens.

An HL-A match and MLC nonreactivity indicate compatibility between donor and recipient. Even when this compatibility is determined, immunosuppression is necessary before and after grafting to prevent rejection.

IMMUNOSUPPRESSION

In leukemia patients high-dose cyclophosphamide therapy followed by total body irradiation with 1000 rads is utilized to suppress bone marrow function. In patients with aplastic anemia, high-dose cyclophosphamide therapy is utilized without radiation to achieve suppression. Further secondary therapy with low-dose methotrexate is used following the graft four times a day for 11 days postgraft, and once a week thereafter for three months to prevent rejection. This is unnecessary in twin to twin transplants where secondary suppression is not needed.

The survival of the human graft has been improved with immunosuppressive therapy. However, the results are not satisfactory. Some investigators believe continuation of tissue matching of donor and recipient with less immunosuppression may achieve more satisfactory results. It seems that the survival of the recipient is less dependent on exact tissue matching, transplant source, and choice of immunosuppressive therapy than careful pretransplant assessment and conditioning, and through intensive posttransplant follow-up of the patient by the health care team.

THE PROCEDURE

The bone marrow transplant procedure is composed of two facets. In the first, the donor is taken to surgery and about 10 ml of bone marrow per kilogram of donor weight is removed from the anterior and posterior iliac crests under general anesthesia. An anticoagulant solution is added to the marrow to inhibit clot formation. A culture media is added to the marrow to keep it viable. The marrow is then strained through fine mesh screens to remove bone and fat particles. The marrow is then placed in a plastic bag and taken to the recipient, in whom it will be transfused in a manner similar to a blood transfusion.

The risks faced by the donor undergoing this procedure consist of risks associated with general anesthesia. Hip tenderness is also present for a few days postaspiration. The donor is usually hospitalized for 24 hours following the marrow aspiration.

The second facet of this procedure consists of the transfusion of the donor's marrow into the recipient. The recipient has been in protective isolation and immunosuppressed prior to the transfusion. Total body irradiation frequently takes place right before the transfusion. The patient is given a sedative and antiemetic to reduce the nausea that often accompanies the irradiation procedure. In addition irradiation also causes diarrhea, chills, and fever. The irradiation procedure may take up to four hours, after which the patient is returned to his room to receive the bone marrow transfusion.

The marrow aspirated from the donor and prepared as described earlier is infused into the recipient as soon as possible via an intravenous route. The nurse should observe for respiratory distress, usually resulting from pulmonary overload subsequent to the infusion of a volume of marrow that is too large or too rapid an infusion of marrow bolus. Allergic reactions such as chills, fever, and hives sometimes occur during the procedure. These reactions can be controlled with Benadryl.

Following the transplant, the recipient is without bone marrow function for 10 days to 3 weeks. This is the time that it takes for the new graft to establish. During this period, assessments for signs of sepsis and bleeding must continually occur. In addition, therapeutic measures should be instituted to prevent the transmission of infection and possibility of trauma to the skin and mucous membranes. Platelet transfusions are provided and antibiotic therapy instituted if sepsis is suspected. The use of white cell transfusions is also sometimes necessary.

Mucosistis, mouth discomfort, and eating problems have been noted and associated with chemotherapy and irradiation. Both preventive and therapeutic mouth care such as saline rinses, nystatin mouthwash, and numbing agents are indicated.

If anorexia occurs, the patient should be encouraged to eat small, frequent meals composed of foods he has selected with the assistance of the dietician. An accurate intake and output is essential, including an accurate calorie count. If oral feedings are inadequate to maintain body mass, hyperalimentation fluids are utilized.

Frequent observation of vital signs is essential to assess for the possibility of sepsis. Rectal temperatures should be avoided because rectal irritation, secondary to radiation, is already present, and the use of the rectal thermometer will only increase the irritation. The use of daily sitz bath may limit or prevent irritation. Blood, throat, urine, and stool cultures are also done regularly to monitor for the possibility of sepsis.

The recipient should be observed for petechiae; emesis, stool, and urine should be hematested for early indications of bleeding. Care of the teeth should be provided, however, toothettes are substituted for toothbrushes to prevent gum trauma.

Psychological support should be provided, especially in the immediate post-graft period when generalized malaise is common. A significant other, parent or spouse, can be of great value in this role. The nurse should encourage the recipient to be out of bed and carry out as many daily activities as possible. All procedures should be explained and demonstrated before they are instituted. The recipient will adjust to his condition more rapidly and participate in his care more actively if he has received realistic expectations of outcomes.

REJECTION

Graft versus host rejection occurs in about 70 percent of recipients. This reaction can involve the skin, liver, and gastrointestinal tract and occurs with varying degrees of severity. Skin involvement begins as an itchy erythematous rash. The rash may resolve spontaneously or progress to a sloughing stage similar to a third-degree burn. Liver function abnormalities may be mild or severe. The reaction in the gastrointestinal tract is frequently diarrhea. It may be mild or severe. Sloughing and passage of the gastrointestinal mucosa may follow, making the digestion and absorption of nutrients impossible. In this case hyperalimentation fluids must be initiated.

When a graft versus host reaction occurs, antithymocyte globulin may be utilized. This is given in the thigh and is irritating to the tissues causing muscle pain and swelling. The pain can be reduced with ultrasound treatments. Active or passive exercise of the extremity is useful to reduce stiffness. The use of additional immunosuppression increases the probability of sepsis. Assessment for early cues related to infection development must be even more vigorous. Therapeutic measures taken to insure protective isolation should be reevaluated and maintained. Interstitial pneumonia is a frequent complication in these patients and is their greastest single cause of death.

The course of graft versus host disease can be extensive and complicated by multiple infections. A hospital stay exceeding two to three months is not uncommon.

DISCHARGE

Protective isolation is maintained to a degree even postdischarge. The family and/or patient should be encouraged to locate close to the hospital for at least three months. During this period, the recipient is checked weekly and receives weekly doses of methotrexate. The recipient is allowed to go outside during this period as long as they wear a face mask and stay out of crowds.

After this three-month period, the recipient returns to his home and is followed by his community physician. This member of the health care team as well as community health nurse should be included in communication during the hospital course and participate in discharge planning. Contact with this community component of the health care team is essential postdischarge. The recipient is usually assessed at the transplant site once a year following discharge.

SUMMARY

Bone marrow transplantation has etched itself a place as an acceptable adjunctive therapy for those with leukemia and aplastic anemia. The process is associated with many problems, some of which are life threatening. The nurse caring for donors and recipients of transplants utilizes concepts from immunology, epidemiology, and psychology as well as the nursing process to construct nursing approaches. Contact with the patient should be direct and consistent. The use of a primary nursing model is the administrative strategy of choice.

Transfer Factor

Transfer factor and thymosin have been given to a limited number of immunoincompetent individuals. Reports indicate restoration of immunocompetency in several cases. In addition, this procedure has been utilized to control metastatic carcinoma in several cases.

RECENT DEVELOPMENTS
AND EXPERIMENTS IN IMMUNOLOGY

Antilymphocyte Serum: Antilymphocyte Globulin

Immunosuppression of the T system has been accomplished by the use of antilymphocyte serum; similarily, antilymphocyte globulin has been used to suppress B cell function. These preparations, as well as cytotoxic drugs, have concurrent hazardous effects. The primary use of this type of preparation has been in transplant patients, and the incidence of malignancy has been notably increased in them. Researchers hypothesize that this reaction is due to a reduction in the T system's surveillance mechanism. (This mechanism was discussed in Chapter 2, p. 17.)

One hypothesis regarding the use of specific antigen in antilymphocyte globulin in transplant patients is that the foreign antigen, once absorbed by the recipient, interacts with antigen reactive cells. These antigens are antibody complexes destroyed by the antilymphocyte globulin, which was specific to donor lymphoid cells. The result is suppression of an undesirable immune response. Although this is still a theory and based on animal research, it was used effectively in a case of Wiskott-Aldrich syndrome. It is possible that the explanatory mechanism behind this phenomenon differs from the hypothesis above, but only further research can answer this question.

Antigen-Mediated Lymphokine Release

It also appears that the nonspecific stimulation of macrophages by lymphokines (released following the interaction of recipient T cells with foreign antigen) can result in limitation of conditions such as leprosy. This is a most intriguing concept, although yet unproven. The possibility that unrelated antigens could be used to manage disease holds promise for future clinical application of immunological concepts.

Bacterial Toxins

Other investigators believe that bacterial toxins (Coley's toxins) and preparations such as bacillus of Calmette and Guerin (BCG) are able to assist in the control of tumor growth (either as adjuvants or as macrophage activators). There are many questions yet to be answered. Are the number of tumor cells reduced? Are tumor antigens altered so that they are recognized and destroyed? Or does the preparation act as an adjuvant to the immunological system? This is another broad area of interest with many implications that will undoubtedly be better understood in the future.

BCG

BCG is the bacillus of Calmette and Guerin and is an attenuated form of the living bovine tubercle bacillus. Its use as an agent utilized to immunize humans against tuberculosis has already been discussed. It also has the potential to increase the human host's immune response against tumor-specific antigens. Intralesional injection or direct injection into tumor nodules has resulted in regression of the nodule in melanoma patients. Intradermal injection of BCG at sites remote from the tumor location has been attempted alone and in combination with allogenic cells in the hope of initiating an intensified immune response against tumor cells. Results of recent investigations have been inconsistent, indicating little effect on increasing remission maintenance in acute lymphocytic leukemia.

Administration. BCG is administered by the scarification method and Heaf Gun injection. In the scarification method, a 5X 5-cm area is anesthetized, cleansed with acetone, and permitted to dry. The vaccine in the desired dose is then spread over the prepared area; 10 vertical and 10 horizontal lines are then scratched through the skin layers. The site is kept clean and dry and may initially be covered with sterile telfa for protection.

The Heaf Gun provides for the administration of BCG via multiple punctures. The skin is prepared as in the scarification method. The desired dose of vaccine is then spread over the prepared area and the area injected with the Heaf Gun in the desired pattern. Protection of the area is provided as in the scarification method. Extremities are the injection sites of choice in both methods and the nurse should rotate injection sites according to a predetermined plan.

The Reaction. A local inflammatory response usually occurs in a few hours after the vaccine is administered. Pruritis is expected at this site. The lesion takes about 24 hours to resolve following initial sensitization. Regional nodes may enlarge, a low-grade fever and generalized malaise have been frequently noted. After sensitization, a flare reaction may occur at the sites of previous injections. As sensitivity increases, ulceration, necrosis, and eschar formation can occur at the injection site; 6 to 9 months may be required for resolution if sloughing occurs. This type of sloughing response is thought to be due to delayed hypersensitivity and superinfection of the site with BCG.

The nurse should assess for generalized sepsis and superimposed local infections. Disseminated infections have occurred varying from an influenza-like syndrome to BCG infection of the injection site, lymph nodes, and pleura. Hepatic dysfunction such as mild alteration of liver function tests as well as hepatosplenomegaly and jaundice have been reported. Repeated intralesional injections have resulted in severe hypersensitivity reactions and death has occurred. Intradermal BCG therapy has been associated with less severe and less frequent reactions. No fatalities have been associated with intradermal BCG therapy.

MER

MER is a methanol extraction residue obtained from a phenolized culture of BCG. The administration of MER results in a nonspecific stimulation of the immunological system. The cellular response to antigens, including those of tumor cells, is thought to be affected. MER is active in a nonviable suspension and can be administered without the threat of tubercular infection.

Administration.   MER is administered intradermally. Several intradermal injections of the desired dose are given at least 3-to-4 cm apart. Ulceration occurs at the injection sites after three to four weeks. The injection site should be protected and kept clean and dry. Subsequent injection should be administered on a site rotation schedule.

The Reaction.   As sensitivity develops, induration of the injection site is marked and is thought to represent a delayed-type hypersensitivity reaction. The sites may ulcerate and necrotize. Severe local reactions require therapy with steroid creams and may result in the decision to terminate therapy. Fever and generalized malaise are common following therapy. Symptomatic treatment is indicated when this occurs.

CORYNEBACTERIUM PARVUM

Corynebacterium parvum is another modality used to stimulate a nonspecific intensified immune response and has been administered both intravenously and subcutaneously. *C. parvum* therapy is thought to act synergistically with chemotherapeutic agents to promote tumor regression in patients with carcinoma, sarcoma, and disseminated melanoma.

Administration. Guidelines for the intravenous administration of *C. parvum* are currently under development. Israel suggests the injection of a dose of 2-to-4 mg intravenously in a dilution that will permit its administration in a 30-min period. The nursing assessment of patients receiving this therapy should include all factors representative of a systemic allergic response. Wheezing and hypertension have been associated with *C. parvum* therapy, and chills, fever, nausea, vomiting, and headache of varying time of onset, intensity, and duration also occur. These symptoms tend to decrease with repeated *C. parvum* therapy.

Reaction. The subcutaneous administration of *C. parvum* is often associated with local pain at the injection site. Induration of the site is common; fever and generalized malaise also occur within two to three days. Allergic reactions have not been reported in association with *C. parvum* subcutaneous administration. Secondary infection of the administration site has been noted and can be prevented through the protection of the injection site from environmental contamination and by keeping the area clean and dry.

SUMMARY

Immunotherapy is an adjunct therapy for patients with cancer. The nurse should maintain and expand knowledge related to the various treatment modalities utilized. An understanding of potential complications will permit the identification of nursing implications and allow the nurse to incorporate these diagnostic, therapeutic, and patient education approaches into nursing practice.

ENVIRONMENTAL IMMUNOSUPPRESSION

Physical X-Irradiation

Irradiation can be used to suppress B lymphocytes function as well as that of the yet unsensitized small lymphocytes. The irradiation process suppresses the immunological response and antibody production. However, the effect of irradiation on cells already in contact with antigen is limited. The use of x-irradiation in suppressing the action of the T system has been shown to be of little value.

Chemical

Antihistamines are used to suppress IgE-mediated injury. Histamine, slow-reacting substances (SRS), and chemotactic factor are released from the lung and nasal mucosa subsequent to challenge with specific antigen. Dibutyl cyclic adenosine $3',5'$-monophosphate, and isoproterenol (a beta-adrenergic agent) can in certain doses inhibit IgE-mediated release of these substances. The use of antihistamine appears to be of most value in the treatment of allergic rhinitis.

DISODIUM CROMOGLYCATE

Disodium cromoglycate is a relatively new medication used to manage asthmatic attacks due to either allergic or nonallergic triggers. This substance appears to inhibit the migration of mast cell granules. In essence, it limits mast cell degranulation and the subsequent allergic response.

STEROIDS

Steroids are not lymphocytic in humans, but they do exhibit a well documented antiinflammatory effect. They are used to treat immune-complex-mediated injury, immune cytolysis, delayed hypersensitivity reactions, and anaphylactic-type injuries. In addition, steroids in combination with cytotoxic drugs have been useful in the treatment of certain lymphomas. In attempting to explain the role of steroids in the treatment of lymphomas, it seems researchers have suggested that the malignant lymphocyte is either capable of binding with more corticosteroid or more sensitive to the action of the steroid.

CYTOTOXIC CHEMICAL AGENTS

Our knowledge of the effect of chemical cytotoxic immunosuppressant agents is drawn from animal studies. These studies have indicated that it is possible to prevent antibody responses, to induce immunological tolerance, to suppress IgG formation while prolonging the production of IgM, to augment antibody formation, and to suppress allograft rejection and hypersensitivity reactions. These agents achieve the desired suppression effect best if the small lymphocyte is still unsensitized. The more determined or specific the lymphocyte is prior to antigenic stimulation, the larger the dose of drug necessary to achieve desired effects. In essence, primary responses are more amenable to suppression than secondary responses. There is little information available regarding the side effects of immunosuppressant therapy with cytotoxic agents. At this time, there is evidence to correlate cytotoxic suppression therapy with an increased incidence of malignancy. These agents have only been used for a short period of time, and a great deal of investigation is necessary before definitive statements can be made regarding their use as immunosuppressive agents in the treatment of cytotoxic disease.

ENVIRONMENTAL AND EXTRINSIC CONDITIONS ASSOCIATED WITH DECREASED HOST DEFENSES

The human organism's anatomical and structural defense barriers have frequently been altered and/or depleted with the advent of increasing technology in diagnostic and therapeutic methods, the aggressive chemotherapy protocols, and the large doses of ionizing radiation. In addition, other life-saving devices, such as parenteral nutrition, artificial devices and prostheses, catheters, intravenous therapy, and the extensive use of the antibiotic drugs, have resulted in new infectious diseases due to bacteria, viruses, and fungi. Many of these organisms formerly known as normal flora are now recognized as pathogens. Microorganisms that rarely cause disease in the absence of an obvious altered host defense but are responsible for infectious disease in an altered host are referred to as opportunistic agents.

Opportunistic infectious disease has become a vast area of research in the field of microbiology. It is difficult to summarize the findings thus far, but an attempt will be made to do so in some of the major areas mentioned in the opening statement of this chapter.

Burns

Among the over 2 million patients who are hospitalized each year for burns, more than 11,000 die. Generally, after providing for survival by preventing shock, the next problem faced in the care of the burn patient is that of septicemia. The severity of the infection varies with the depth and area of the burn, and the primary mechanical host defenses can be compromised if the burn involves more than 30 percent of the body surface. Changes following burns include arteriolar constriction with venous stasis, sloughing of epithelial cells, marked abnormalities of the polymorphonuclear cells with decreased intracellular killing and depressed skin reactions. This later may account for the inadequate T-cell-mediated graft versus host reaction in these patients. Skin grafts are accepted more readily by burn patients than by normal persons.

The immunoglobulin levels are also decreased, and the number of circulating plasma cells falls. Immunoglobulin levels are probably the lowest two days post-trauma. At the end of the first week IgM and IgD levels return to normal. IgG, IgA, and IgE levels return to normal at about the end of the second week.

Bacteria gain entry via the traumatized skin and other affected routes usually resistant to invasion, e.g., the respiratory and gastrointestinal tracts. Antibiotics have effectively reduced streptococcal and staphylococcal infections. The problems for these patients are created by common environmental organisms, e.g.,

Pseudomonas aeruginosa, Clostridium tetani, Candida albicans, Streptococcus pneumoniae. Cytomegalovirus and *Herpes homines* also occur, but less frequently.

Infection can be reduced by rigid environmental control. However, other measures can be helpful in some cases. Passive immunization with hyperimmune plasma or gamma globulin has been used effectively in preventing overwhelming infections. Another passive immunization being used is hyperimmune Pseudomonas serum. It seems that these preparations are capable of facilitating the function of the polymorphonuclear cells.

Operative Procedures

Infection is a well-recognized complication of surgical intervention. About 1000 persons die each year from postoperative hospital-associated infections. In 1964, an estimated 9.5 percent of all surgical wounds resulted in posthospital infections. This suggests that a possible 1.5 million postoperative surgical infections occur each year.

Both surgery and anesthesia have a depressive effect on immunological function, although the exact mechanisms are not well understood. Pathogens such as coagulase-positive *S. aureus* and group A beta-hemolytic streptococcus are the most common sources of infection in these patients.

Among the opportunists known to precipitate infections in surgical wounds is *Staphylococcus epidermidis.* In a study from 1957 to 1964 in one hospital, *S. epidermidis* was identified as the causative agent in 53 to 1200 patients with postoperative infections. Some of these infections result in septicemia. *Bacillus subtiles,* Alcaligenes fecalis, and others have also been incriminated.

Candida albicans, a fungus, has become a prominent problem in patients receiving prophylactic antibiotic therapy. Fungal organisms are responsible for infection predominantly in patients having abdominal and cardiac surgery.

Stressors that Mechanically Alter Local Defenses

Agents known to stress local defenses are needles, catheters, intravenous infusions, and hyperalimentation.

Needles penetrate the skin, making a portal of entry available to organisms normally kept out by skin barriers. The larger the bore of the needle, the greater the possibility of infection, a principle that applies to injections as well as to intravenous catheters. The organisms most frequently associated with infection in these cases are *S. epidermidis,* bacteroides, C. albicans, *Pseudomonas,* Criptococcus, and Mimeae.

Urinary catheters establish a new portal of entry and provide a potential area of stasis as well as an excellent environment for bacterial growth. Contaminated equipment is a frequent source of bacterial invasion.

Hyperalimentation supplements have long been associated with a high level of infection. This could be due to the large bore of the catheter as well as the concomitant decrease in endogenous flora, which allows the pathogens to take over. The debilitated condition of these patients is another variable that must be considered. *C. albicans* is a potential enemy of these patients.

Last but not least in this area of potential environmental stressors is the possibility of fluid contamination. Commercially available fluids are usually under rigid quality control protocols that limit contamination; however, there have been reports of contamination resulting from inadequate quality control. Also, fluids are often contaminated when they are opened, when additives are mixed with the fluids, or when outdated fluids are used.

Prostheses

Cardiac valves, shunt devices, and vascular replacement prostheses all are associated with an increased risk of infection. These foreign materials all provide an entry route for bacteria either at the time of installation or later as a site of stasis and/or obstruction. The common offending organisms are *S. aureus, S. epidermides,* and Staphylococcus albus.

Respiratory Therapy

The increased use of inhalation therapy and respirators for life support has provided another potential area for infection development. Usually the tubing, reservoirs, or nebulizers are the sources of contamination. These pieces of equipment must be frequently and fastidiously cleaned, while in use and before therapy is initiated.

Drugs

The increased use of drug therapy, i.e., antibiotics, antineoplastics, and immunosuppressive agents, has led to an increased incidence of nonpathogenic infections in those receiving these medications. The general effect of these medications on host defenses in summarized in Table 6.

Antibiotics alter the normal flora of the skin, mucous membranes, and gastrointestinal tract. Suppression of the flora of the gastrointestinal tract has resulted in an increased incidence of infections due to the fungi *C. albicans*. Broad-spectrum antibiotics affect phagocytosis and mobility of the leukocyte. Antimicrobial drugs can alter the pH of body fluids, resulting in vitamin deficiencies and Candida proliferation. Most patients recover quickly from Candida infections when the antibiotic therapy is discontinued.

CORTICOSTEROIDS

Corticosteroids have many uses, and the mechanism by which they function is not fully understood. They interfere with the inflammatory response by altering the activities of lymphocytes. There is a decrease of both T and B cells in the circulation of patients treated with these medications. If alternate-day therapy is utilized the lymphocytopenia and monocytopenia is transitory, thus this schedule is the method of choice. However, alternate-day therapy has not always been successful in continued suppression of malignant and hematological diseases. Long-term therapy with these agents is associated with infections due to bacteria, fungi, viruses, and parasites. Herpes infections during steroid therapy have resulted in superinfections and fatal pneumonia, especially in patients receiving cardiac and renal transplants.

ANTINEOPLASTIC DRUGS AND RADIATION

Therapy with antineoplastic drugs and radiation results in immunosuppression. These therapies share an alkylating effect on the cell during mitosis. They affect all cells but especially those which

TABLE 6 The Effect of Medications on Most Defenses

MEDICATION	EFFECT
Antibiotics	Changes normal bacterial flora of the gastrointestinal tract, skin, mucous membranes, and respiratory tract.
	May result in growth of resistant strains and increased fungal growth.
	May alter serum immunoglobulins.
Glucocorticosteroids	Suppression of the inflammatory response.
	Depression of the reticuloendothelial system.
	Depression of the lymphoid system.
Antimetabolites and irradiation	Bone marrow depression.
	Depression of the reticuloendothelial system.
	Inhibition of antibody formation.
	Injury to other cells, especially rapidly growing cells.

proliferate rapidly. The suppressant effect is dose related and also dependent on the amount of time the therapy is utilized. Patients receiving these preparations are prone to infections from gram-negative organisms, viruses, and fungi. When viral infections occur, they seem to be related to reactivation of a latent infection. Most infections are systemic and have visceral involvement.

Treatment of Opportunistic Infections

Approaches to therapeutic intervention would by nature fall into the categories of preventions and treatment. Infection control committees in institutions can set guidelines, further research, and provide lists of items of potential danger. All items in the patient's external environment must be reviewed in light of this potential for the immunoincompetent patient.

Other therapeutic interventions can take the form of replacing the deficient blood components, e.g., transfusions of granulocytes, transfer factor, bone marrow transplants. Antimicrobial agents are available for some of the opportunistic infections, while many more are being tested and have not yet been approved for general use.

There is a recognized and well-developed role for a nurse in the area of epidemiology. The nurse epidemiologist plays a major role in the identification of variables associated with infection control. One of the functions of the nurse epidemiologist includes an assessment to track down, treat, and eradicate infections. The nurse epidemiologist consults with the health team and plans for the proper procedural techniques to prevent and control the infection. In addition, the role of the nurse epidemiologist includes planning and implementing educational programs for staff, patients, and family members. Lastly, the nurse epidemiologist assists with and initiates research designs.

Much is known about the control and prevention of infectious diseases, but there is a great deal still to be learned. Every nurse, not just the nurse epidemiologist, must be keenly aware of the epidemiology of infectious agents as well as the mechanism by which they can be controlled. The priority will always be the prevention of disease through the promotion of health.

SUMMARY

Many microorganisms formerly considered normal flora and in a broad sense nonpathogenic to man have now been proven responsible for acute and sometimes fatal infectious diseases to the compromised immunoincompetent patient. Factors contributing to this breakdown in host defense range from advances in technology, life-prolonging/saving techniques and equipment, radiation therapy and drugs. This is a new and challenging frontier for research.

SUGGESTED READINGS

Immunizations

American Academy of Pediatrics: Report of the Committee on Infectious Disease. Evanston, Ill., 1975

Arenstein MS et al: Prevention of meningococcal disease by Group C polysaccharide vaccine. N Eng J Med 282:417–420, 1970

Ashcroft MT et al: A seven year field of two typhoid vaccines in Guyana. Lancet 2:1056–58, 1967

Austin SM et al: Joint reactions in children vaccinated against rubella. Am J Epidemiol 95:53–56, 1972

Balagtas RC et al: Treatment of pertussis with pertussis immune globulin. J Pediatr 79:203–208, 1971

Baratta RO et al: Measles (rubeola) in previously immunized children. Pediatrics 46:397–402, 1970

Bellanti JA, Arenstein MS: Mechanisms of immunity to virus infection. Pediatr Clin N Am 11:558–567, 1964

Brandt BL et al: Antibody responses to meningococcal polysaccharide vaccines. Infect Immunol 8:590, 1973

Brooks VB et al: Mode of action of tetanus toxin. Nature 175:150–151, 1955

Bunyak EB, Hillman MR: Live attenuated mumps virus vaccine. I. Vaccine development. Proc Soc Exp Bio Med 123:768–775, 1966

Chin J et al: Field evaluation of a respiratory syncytial virus vaccine and a trivalent parainfluenza virus vaccine in a pediatric population. Am J Epidemiol 89:449–463, 1969

Cooper L: Rubella: a preventable cause of birth defects. In Birth Defects: Original Article Series, vol 4, no 7, 23–35, 1968

Dufour FD: Correlation between the mumps virus skin test antigen and cutaneous delayed hypersensitivity. J Pediatr 81:742–746, 1972

Edsall G: Passive immunization. Pediatrics 32:444–456, 1963

Edsall G et al: Excessive use of tetanus toxoid boosters. JAMA 202:17–19, 1967

Eickhoff TC: Committee on Infectious Disease: rationale and recommendations. J Infect Dis 123:446–453, 1971

Fulginiti VA et al: Altered reactivity to measles virus. Amer J Dis Child 115: 671–676, 1968

Fuller RM, Ellerbeck W: Tetanus prophylaxis. JAMA 174:1–4, 1960

Gellis SS et al: A study of the prevention of mumps orchitis by gamma globulin. Am J Med Sci 210:661–664, 1945

Horstmann DM et al: Rubella: the challenge of its control. J Infect Dis 123: 640–654, 1971

Karliner JS, Beleval GS: Incidence of reactions following administration of antirabies anti-serum: study of 526 cases. JAMA 193:359–362, 1965

Kemp CH, Beneson AS: Smallpox immunization in the United States. JAMA 194:61–66, 1962

Kemp CH et al: Smallpox vaccination of eczema patients with a strain of attenuated live vaccinia (CVI-78). Pediatrics 42:980–985, 1968

Kenrick P, Elderling G: A study of active immunization against pertussis. Am J Hyg 29:133–139, 1939

Koprowski H: Live poliomyelitis virus vaccines: present status and problems for the future. JAMA 178:1151–1155, 1961

Krugman S: Present status of measles and rubella immunization in the United States: a medical progress report. J Pediatr 78:1–16, 1971

Krugman S et al: Viral hepatitis, Type B (MS-2 strain): studies on active immunization. JAMA 217:41–45, 1971

Larson HE et al: Inadvertent rubella virus vaccination during pregnancy. New Engl J Med 284:870–873, 1971

MacLead CM: Prevention of pneumococcal pneumonia by immunization with specific capsular polysaccharides. In Mudd S (ed): Infectious Agents and Host Reactions. Philadelphia, Saunders, 1970

Mel DM et al: Studies on vaccination against bacillary dysentery. Four oral immunizations with live monotypic and combined vaccines. Bull WHO 39:375-380, 1968

Mensen MA et al: Rubella viruria in a 29 year old woman with congenital rubella. Lancet 2:797, 1971

Meyer HM, Parkman P: Rubella vaccination: a review of practical experience. JAMA 215:613-619, 1971

Monto AS: Frequency of arthralgia in women receiving one of three rubella vaccines. Arch Int Med 126:635-639, 1970

Plotkin SA et al: Oral polio virus vaccination in newborn African infants: the inhibitory effect on breast feeding. Amer J Dis Child III:27-30, 1966

Rees RJW: BCG vaccination in mycobacteria infections. Brit Med Bull 25: 183-196, 1969

Sabin AB: Is there an exceedingly small risk associated with oral polio virus vaccine? JAMA 183:268-271, 1963

Smith CB et al: Protective effect of antibody to parainfluenza Type I virus. New Engl J Med 275:1145-1152, 1966

Standfast AFB: Pertussis, typhoid-paratyphoid and cholera vaccines. Brit Med J Bull 25:189-194, 1969

Stollerman GH: Prospects for a vaccine against Group A. Streptococci: the problem of the immunology of the M proteins. Arth Rheum 10:245-250, 1967

Terry L: The association of cases of poliomyelitis with the use of Type III oral poliomyelitis vaccines: a technical report. U.S. Department of Health, Education and Welfare, September 20, 1962

Waldman RH et al: Influenza antibody response following aerosol administration of inactivated virus. Amer J Epidemiol 91:575-584, 1970

Wallace RB et al: Joint symptoms following an area-wide rubella immunization campaign—report of a survey. Amer J Pub Health 62:658-661, 1972

Suppression of the Immune Response

Abrahams S et al: Inhibition of the immune response by 75 antibody, mechanism and site of action. J Exp Med 137:870, 1973

Bast RC et al: BCG and cancer (second of two parts). N Engl J Med 290: 1458-1469, 1974

Brown JAK et al: BCG vaccination of children against leprosy: first results of a trial in Uganda. Br Med J 1:7, 1966

Coley WB: Current enigmas in cancer reasearch. In Old LJ, Boyse EA (eds): The Harvey Lectures, Series 67. New York, Academic, 1973

Freda VJ: The control of Rh disease. In Good RA, Fisher DW (eds): Immunobiology. Stanford, Conn, Sinauer Assoc, Inc, 1971, p 266

Harris JE, Sinkovics JG: Suppression of the Human Immune Response in the Immunology of Malignant Disease. St. Louis, Mosby, 1970, p 1973

Israel L et al: Brief communication: daily intravenous infusions of Corynebac-

terium parvum in twenty patients with disseminated cancer. J Natl
Cancer Inst 55:29–33, July 1975

Kaliner M et al: Immunological release of chemical mediators from human
nasal polyps. N Engl J Med 289:277, 1973

Lance EM et al: Antilymphocyte serum. Adv Immunol 17:2, 1973

Lawrence HS: Transfer factor. Adv Immunol 11:195, 1969

McCalla J: Immunotherapy: concepts and nursing implications. Nurs Clin
N Am 11:1:49–57, 1976

Miller ME: Uses and abuses of gamma globulin. In Good RA, and Fisher DW
(eds): Immunobiology. Stanford, Conn, Sinauer Assoc, Inc, 1971

Orr TSC: Current review: Mode of action of disodium cromoglycate. Current
Titles in Immunological Transplantation. Allergy 1:217, 1973

Pross HF, Eidinger D: Antigenic competition: a review of non-specific antigen-
induced suppression. Adv Immunol 18:133, 1974

Rowley DA et al: Specific suppression of all mediated immune responses.
Transplant Proc 1:580, 1969

Schwartz R (ed): Proceedings of the symposium on immunosuppressive drugs.
Fed Proc 26:879, 1967

Schwartz R: Therapeutic strategy in clinical immunology. N Engl J Med 280:
367, 1969

Schwitter G, Beach J: Bone marrow transplantation in children. Nurs Clin N
Am 11:1:49–57, 1976

Scott MT: Corynebacterium parvum as an immunotherapeutic anti-cancer
agent. Semin Oncol 1:376–378, 1974

Skinner MD, Schwartz RS: Immunosuppressive therapy. N Engl J Med 287:
221–281, 1972

Smith RT: Possibilities and problems of immunological intervention in cancer.
N Engl J Med 287:439, 1972

Thomas ED et al: Bone marrow transplantation using matched sibling donors.
Transplantation Proc 6:110–116, 1974

Thomas ED et al: Bone marrow transplantation (Part I). N Engl J Med
292:832, 1975

Thomas ED et al: Bone marrow transplantation (Part II). N Engl J Med
292:895, 1975

Van Rood JJ, Eernisse JG: The detection of transplant antigens in leukocytes.
Prog Surg 7:217, 1967

Yron I et al: Immunotherapeutic studies in mice with the methanol-extrac-
tion residue (MER) fraction of BCG: solid tumors. Conference on the
use of BCG in Therapy of Cancer. National Cancer Institute Monograph
39:33–35, Dec. 1973

**Environmental and Extrinsic Conditions
Associated with Decreased Host Defenses**

Alexander JW, Fisher MW: Immunization against pseudomonas in infection
after thermal injury. J Infect Dis 130:152, 1974

Alexander JW, Meakins JL: A physiologic basis for the development of
opportunistic infection in man. Ann Surg 176:273, 1972

Arthurson G et al: Changes in immunoglobulin levels in severely burned patients. Lancet 1:546, 1969

Balch HH: Septicemia in burned patients. Ann NY Acad Sci 150:991–1000, 1968

Casson PR et al: Delayed hypersensitivity states of burned patients. Surg Forum 17:268, 1966

Lauter B: Opportunistic infections. Heart Lung 5(4):601–606, 1976

Law EJ et al: Experience with systemic candidiasis in the burned patient. J Trauma 12:543–552, 1972

Liksky BY: Microbiology and post-op infections. AORN J 19:37–52, 1974

Meakins J: Body's response to infection. AORN J 22:37–51, 1974

Papageorgiou P: Impairment of natural defenses (the compromised host): introduction. Pediatr Ann 5:50–51, 1976

Papageorgiou P: Impairment of natural defenses. I. Exogenous causes, mechanisms and opportunistic infection. Pediatr Ann 5:55–83, 1976

Prier JE, Friedman H (eds): Opportunistic Pathogens. Baltimore, University Park Press, 1974

Sherman RT: The prevention and treatment of tetanus in the burn patient. Surg Clin N Am 50:1277–81, 1970

Stiehm ER, Fulginiti VA: Immunologic disorders in infants and children. Philadelphia, Saunders, 1973

Index

151